Clinicians' Guide to Pain

Clinicians' Guide to Pain

T.W.I. Lovel
FRCP
Consultant Physician in Palliative Medicine,
St. Benedict's Hospice, Monkwearmouth Hospital,
Sunderland, UK

and

W.U. Hassan
MB, FRCP (Ed), MD (Newcastle)
Consultant Rheumatologist,
Sunderland Royal Hospital,
Sunderland, UK
and
Honorary Clinical Lecturer,
Department of Medicine,
University of Newcastle upon Tyne, UK

A member of the Hodder Headline Group
LONDON · SYDNEY · AUCKLAND
Co-published in the United States of America by
Oxford University Press Inc., New York

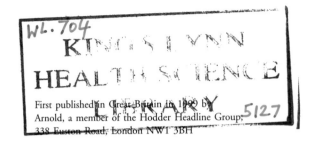
First published in Great Britain in 1999 by
Arnold, a member of the Hodder Headline Group,
338 Euston Road, London NW1 3BH

http://www.arnoldpublishers.com

Co-published in the United States of America by
Oxford University Press Inc.,
198 Madison Avenue, New York, NY10016
Oxford is a registered trademark of Oxford University Press

Whilst the advice and information in this book are believed to be true and
accurate at the date of going to press, neither the authors nor the publisher can
accept any legal responsibility or liability for any errors or omissions that may be
made. In particular (but without limiting the generality of the preceding
disclaimer) every effort has been made to check drug dosages; however, it is still
possible that errors have been missed. Furthermore, dosage schedules are
constantly being revised and new side-effects recognized. For these reasons the
reader is strongly urged to consult the drug companies' printed instructions before
administering any of the drugs recommended in this book.

British Library Cataloguing in Publication Data
A catalogue record for this book is available from the British Library

Library of Congress Cataloging-in-Publication Data
A catalog record for this book is available from the Library of Congress

ISBN 0 340 74097 3

1 2 3 4 5 6 7 8 9 10

Commissioning Editor: Jo Koster
Production Editor: Rada Radojicic
Production Controller: Priya Gohil

Typeset in 11/13 Adobe Garamond by Photoprint, Torquay, Devon
Printed and bound in Great Britain by the Alden Press, Oxford

What do you think about this book? Or any other Arnold title?
Please send your comments to feedback.arnold@hodder.co.uk

Contents

Preface

Pain is the commonest symptom of patients with rheumatic diseases and of those with cancer. It is an unpleasant, subjective feeling, the intensity of which varies from a mild ache to severe persistent pain. Painful musculoskeletal disorders constitute a major bulk of the family physician's workload, while the pain of cancer is dreaded by all and is frequently not well managed.

The first section of this book deals with the management of cancer pain. There is discussion of the pathophysiology of cancer pain, including neural transmission and pain perception at the spinal and the cortical level. The chapters on cancer pain deal with the particular problems of pain in solid viscera, bone, nerves, bowel and bladder. The need to reach a precise diagnosis is emphasized and the usefulness and drawbacks of all medications currently used is reviewed. Throughout, the emphasis is on evidence based medicine; for too long palliative care has been largely pragmatic and empirical with few well designed randomized controlled trials to justify the drugs and dosages used. Such evidence is still lacking in many instances, but wherever possible peer reviewed papers are quoted to support the advice given.

The section of rheumatology initially deals with the pathophysiology of rheumatic pain. There is a brief introduction in each chapter, followed by a discussion on the management of common rheumatic disorders such as rheumatoid arthritis, osteoarthritis, low back pain and osteoporotic vertebral crush fractures. There is also discussion on the role of physiotherapy and occupational therapy in the management of rheumatic pain. Finally, there is a chapter on procedures, including articular and periarticular injections.

A basic knowledge of pain management is of paramount importance to all clinicians. This book is particularly intended for those dealing with cancer and rheumatic pain such as family physicians. It will also be of relevance to doctors in training and allied health professionals, including physiotherapists, occupational therapists and specialist nurses dealing with cancer and rheumatic pain.

T.W.I. Lovel
W.U. Hassan

Acknowledgement

We are grateful to the librarians and medical photographers of the Sunderland Royal Hospital who have made our task so much easier in compiling this book. We particularly thank all our colleagues, and most of all our patients from whom we have learned greatly.

Part One:
Cancer Pain

The pain of cancer

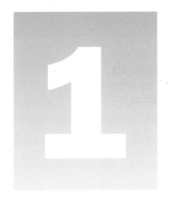

Nothing arouses a livelier fear of pain to come than the word 'cancer'. It is widely known in every community that cancer causes pain and it is a common misbelief that this pain is excruciating and cannot be relieved by any method. So great is the fear that many patients who are otherwise well composed and calm about their illness and its incurable nature none the less dread the pain that is bound to come. In large series of patients it has been shown that about 80% with cancer will experience pain, and of these between 40 and 50% will suffer severe pain.

At the outset of caring for such a patient and in dealing with his or her relatives, it is therefore important to verbalize these fears if possible, to bring them into the open, to examine them and to convince the patient in a rational but not too enthusiastic or hearty a way that they are misplaced. Pain **can** be treated. Pain can be anticipated and prevented. And most pains are not difficult to relieve totally and permanently. Compared with other symptoms, such as breathlessness, pain is in fact one of the easier problems that we normally encounter. Reassurance on this is therefore of the utmost importance long before treatment is commenced.

It is also important to realize that physical pain is only a part of the whole. Patients frequently experience profound emotional pain caused by the diagnosis, by their perceived mortality, by fear and by grieving at their expected bereavement from their family and friends. Patients may also experience quite profound anger, particularly if they feel that they are being cheated of an important part of their life. They feel acutely that life is unfair, that they have done nothing to suffer such a fate, that with better treatment or earlier diagnosis the outcome would have been different, and that they deserve better. There can be a social component to this pain as they contemplate their loss of earning power, a feeling that they should have provided better for their family in financial or social terms, that their relatives are unsympathetic or uncaring or even that they are anticipating their death in order to share out their worldly assets. Finally, there is sometimes a deep spiritual pain that their life has been meaningless, that their God has deserted them or is cruelly indifferent to their suffering. This

Table 1.1

Evaluation of pain in cancer

Believe the patient's report of pain
Initiate discussions about pain
Evaluate the severity of the patient's pain
Take a detailed history of the pain
Evaluate the psychological state of the patient
Perform a careful physical examination
Order and personally review any necessary investigations
Consider alternative methods of pain relief
Monitor the results of treatment

Reprinted with permission from R.G. Twycross, *Pain Relief in Advanced Cancer*, Churchill Livingstone, 1994 (after WHO, 1994).

induces a feeling of hopelessness and despair. All these aspects should be borne in mind when evaluating cancer pain (Table 1.1).

The four components of pain – the physical, the emotional, the social and the spiritual – have been summarized by Dame Cicely Saunders in the concept of total pain. Not every patient has all aspects of it, but many have two or three components and some do have all four. All must be addressed. The relief of physical suffering is only the first small step in dealing with the totality of the pain that the patient is feeling. Derek Doyle has written that no man can deal with his emotions if he is racked by physical pain, but doctors and nurses delude themselves if they believe that the relief of such physical suffering is the be all and end all of palliative care.

It should not be assumed that because a patient has pain and has cancer that the two are necessarily causally related. Patients may have a variety of pains quite unconnected with their malignant disease or with the treatment they are receiving for it. Such patients are often elderly and have a variety of different co-existing pathologies. They may have advanced and painful arthritis, angina, a peptic ulcer or diverticulitis. Treatment of these pains as though all derive from the cancer will produce understandably poor results. In a series of consecutive patients admitted to the hospice in Oxford for pain relief, Twycross & Fairfield (1982) found that in 22% the cause of the pain had nothing whatever to do with the patients' cancer, the treatment or direct results such as bedsores (Table 1.2). Therefore, very careful analysis of the cause of each pain that the patient feels is mandatory if an accurate diagnosis, and therefore precise treatment, is to be achieved.

Pain, cancer and the patient

Everybody knows that cancer causes pain. The inevitability of pain and the inexorable decline towards death are two reasons why this group of diseases

	Number of pains	Number of patients
Caused by cancer		
Bone	58	31
Nerve compression	56	31
Soft tissue infiltration	35	31
Visceral involvement	33	31
Raised intracranial pressure	2	2
Myopathy	2	2
Subtotal	186 (61%)	91
Related to cancer or debility		
Muscle spasm	14	11
Constipation	11	11
Capsulitis of shoulder	4	4
Lymphoedema	4	3
Bedsore	1	1
Postherpetic neuralgia	1	1
Pulmonary embolus	1	1
Bladder spasm (catheter)	1	1
Subtotal	37 (12%)	33
Related to treatment		
Postoperative	8	7
Colostomy	2	2
Nerve block	2	1
Postoperative adhesions	1	1
Postradiation fibrosis	1	1
Oesophageal	1	1
Subtotal	15 (5%)	12
Concurrent disorders		
Myofascial	24	12
Spondylosis	12	11
Osteoarthritis	4	3
Ischial tuberosity	2	1
Migraine	2	2
Sacroiliac	1	1
Miscellaneous	20	15
Subtotal	65 (22%)	45
Total	303 (100%)	100

Table 1.2
Causes of pain in 100 cancer pain patients

Reprinted with permission from R.G. Twycross, *Pain Relief in Advanced Cancer*, Churchill Livingstone, 1994 (after Twycross & Fairfield, 1982).

more than any other is feared and dreaded by the general public. Even now when modern palliative methods have been available for some, if not all, patients for at least 30 years it is still very widely believed that the diagnosis of disseminated cancer means terrible and unalieviated suffering. Every patient and his or her relatives know of somebody – a relative, a person at work, a neighbour in the next street – who, as they say, 'died screaming'.

Case report

A 59-year-old man was found to have lung cancer with bony metastases, and was visited at home by a palliative care consultant to discuss his future management. He was symptom free and resigned to his diagnosis and prognosis. He was comfortable, relaxed, almost blasé and was planning with his wife where they would go, and which relatives they would meet during the time that he had left. All seemed tranquil until the doctor asked 'Have you known anyone else who has had this sort of problem'? The man sat bolt upright in bed and shouted 'Yes'! He then described how not long after they had been married his wife's mother had developed carcinoma of breast. It had progressed very rapidly with widespread bony metastases and they had nursed her to the end of her life. Clearly, pain relief had been very poor and at the recollection of it both of them wept bitterly. The unspoken memories crowded in upon them and they then admitted that they were regarding the husband's future with great fear and terror, for they had seen how a patient died of cancer and imagined that exactly the same suffering was in store for him.

Such beliefs are widespread. In a telephone survey of 1004 Americans, Bostrom (1997) found that 46% had experienced severe pain at some time, 24% had had severe pain in the previous two months and 92% of them said it was 'part of life'. Of those surveyed, 66% had taken nothing for pain the last time they had experienced it, 20% had taken some form of analgesic, and 71% had avoided the doctor, though whether because of the financial cost or because of the serious diagnosis that might be revealed was not clear. Only 18% said that they would take medication quickly if they had pain, 46% said they would avoid medication unless the pain got bad and 35% said they would avoid medication unless the pain was really unbearable. Eighty-two per cent said they felt that it was too easy to become reliant on analgesics and almost the same number (72%) felt that if they took pain killers too readily they would not work when they really needed them. Seventy-seven per cent preferred natural methods before drugs and 79% felt that if one thought about pain it hurt more.

Grond et al. (1996) conducted a prospective evaluation in 2266 cancer patients who had been referred to a pain service in Germany. Seventy-seven per cent of these rated the average pain intensity as being severe or worse, even though 92% were already being treated with analgesics or co-analgesics. A total of 4542 anatomically distinct pain syndromes were identified in these patients. Thirty per cent of them had only one pain, 39% had two pains and 31% had three or more pains. In this series, pain was most frequently localized in the lower back, the abdomen, the thorax and lower limbs. Patients with cancer of the breast had the greatest number of pain syndromes, particularly with bony pain. In 269 of the patients (9%) the pains were entirely unrelated to either the cancer or the treatment for it. These pains were in bone (4%), soft tissue (2%), visceral (1%), neuropathic (3%) and causes unknown (1%).

Twycross, Harcourt and Bergl (1996) similarly found that out of 111 patients admitted to hospice with cancer and with pain there were 370 pains present with a median score of 3 pains per patient. Eighty-five per cent of the patients had more than one pain and 40% had four or more pains. The cancer was directly responsible for only half of these pains and the more severe pain definitely interfered with activity and the enjoyment of life. The pains were scored by the Wisconsin brief pain inventory (BPI) weekly for four weeks. Seventy-six patients were able to complete two questionnaires but only 46 achieved completion of all five of them. After two weeks, 97% of patients had obtained 50% relief of pain and 46% had achieved 90–100% relief. The pains were reduced from a median 3 to 1.5 and the number of patients with four or more pains fell from 40% to 20%. The intensity of the pain also fell. Twenty per cent of patients were completely pain free, though 30% still had severe pain. The authors commented that the Wisconsin brief pain inventory was not brief enough for routine use in clinical practice.

Ward *et al.* (1993) reported that patients do not use analgesics readily and do not accurately report pain. They studied 270 patients who completed a questionnaire about their concerns. The main conclusion was that 'good' patients don't complain. Certainly, many doctors find that patients are not reliable witnesses to the pain they are experiencing, wishing either to appear brave or not to admit the severity of their illness. They are also all too ready to please the doctor by asserting that their treatment has been completely successful when this is often not the case.

How then are we to obtain an objective measurement of pain and of the success of pain treatments? This problem has bedevilled both research workers and clinicians dealing with pain for many years. A variety of tools have been elaborated which aim to give some numerical rating and some semi-objective basis to what is essentially a highly subjective experience. The various pain score tools have been recently reviewed by De Conno *et al.* (1994). They studied 53 patients with chronic cancer pain and administered to them five tools for pain measurement. These were a visual analogue scale

(VAS), a numerical rating scale (NRS), a verbal rating scale (VRS), a pain questionnaire derived from the McGill pain inventory (PRI), and an integrated pain score which was originated in Milan (IPS). All patients used all five scores before and after each change in treatment. The three simpler scales correlated better both with the clinical picture and with the opinions of doctors and nurses than did the more complicated ones.

Choiniere and Amsel (1996) proposed a novel visual analogue thermometer (VAT) for measuring pain intensity. This replaced the normal visual scale and consisted of a red band which the patient pushed across a scale to indicate the intensity of the pain. The distance the red band had travelled in millimetres was then measured on the back of the instrument. Patients preferred this to the VAS and good correlation was found between the VAT and the McGill pain questionnaire. The authors felt that this tool was valid, accurate and useful both for clinical practice and for trial work.

Whatever tool is chosen must be simple (not oppressive to the patient, relatives or professionals), well validated and give some numerical accuracy. It is becoming increasingly important to score pain for the best clinical outcome, for audit and research, and for objective evidence of how both individuals and groups of patients have fared if the work done by their doctors and nurses is questioned after the patients have died. It then becomes possible for local, regional and national standards for cancer pain management to be elaborated.

In a vast study of patients and staff over 3 years Bookbinder *et al.* (1996) used a programme of continuous quality improvement (CQI) which aimed to develop a uniform pain management programme throughout the clinical practice of the hospitals involved. This programme put up a 'red flag' against unrelieved pain, made information about analgesics available to clinicians, gave patients opportunities to report pain freely, allowed policies and methods to evolve, and monitored the success of the standards that had been set. Based on experience from using this programme, the patient's daily temperature, pulse and respiration chart was modified to include a pain score and the accessibility of the relief prescribed for it. A huge staff education programme was undertaken with focus groups being set up to 'Tell it how it is'. Yet in spite of all this effort the worst pain reported by a patient was still 7.7 out of 10 at the end of this trial. The percentage of pain relief experienced by patients actually fell from 82% to 78% and the pain intensity experienced in the last 24 hours of life rose from 5.0 to 5.7, which indicated that data were being collected but not acted upon. It was found that patients often reported higher satisfaction scores and yet were still in pain. The authors commented that clinicians need to respond to a pain chart with the same rapidity and urgency as they would to a chart showing a pyrexia.

Cleeland *et al.* (1994) reported the Eastern Co-operative Oncology Group (ECOG) study of pain and treatment of pain in 1308 outpatients. Sixty-seven per cent had pain or had taken analgesics in the week before the study, and 36% had pain sense enough to impair function. Forty-two per cent of those in pain rated their analgesia as inadequate. Ethnic minorities were three times more likely to have inadequate analgesia, as were the old, those still performing well, and those with pain not attributed to cancer.

Banning, Sjogren and Henriksen (1991) also studied cancer pain in an outpatient clinic. Two hundred patients were referred and of these 172 patients had pain on motion, 144 had pain at rest and 124 had pains which interrupted sleep. After 1–2 weeks of treatment the benefits could be evaluated in 131 patients. Of these, 35 out of 108 patients had pain on motion, 83 out of 123 had pain at rest and 20/92 had pain interrupting sleep. The overall pain relief reported in these 131 patients was: no relief 14, slight 17, moderate 25, considerable 65, complete 10. These workers used a whole range of drug treatments, adjuvants, non-neurolytic nerve blockade, epidural opioids and combinations of these plus psychological intervention and social worker assistance when required.

The difficulty of measuring pain accurately is compounded by the placebo effect. This was elegantly reviewed by Patrick Wall (1992) in an editorial which pointed out why professionals so dislike it. He wrote that placebos have an aura of quackery about them, that they are seen as tiresome and expensive artefacts, that mentioning the placebo effect is taken as a hostile questioning of the validity of the logic of a therapy and that the placebo shakes our belief in the reliability of our sensory experience. He quoted examples where patients had been given a double-blind trial of angina treated with sham operations with ligation of the internal mammary artery. There was no difference between the two groups when only one of them had actually had an operation performed. In most of the patients in each group there was a marked improvement in angina and exercise tolerance and even in their ECG trace. These improvements lasted at least six months. Another trial examined the effects of ultrasound on the pain and swelling following the extraction of wisdom teeth. The ultrasound machine was equally effective whether or not it was turned on, provided that both patient and therapist believed that it was emitting ultrasound. Wall pointed out that not only is pain reduced by the placebo treatment but also that it is extremely active in reducing swelling. Far from believing that all placebo responders are neurotic, or that there is a fixed fraction (33%) of the population who will always respond to a placebo, or that some people are constant placebo responders, Wall pointed out that McQuay, Carroll and Moore (1996) in an analysis of five randomized controlled trials containing 525 patients showed that the proportion varied widely. Between

7 and 38% of patients on a placebo obtained 10% of the maximum possible relief and 16% obtained more than 50% of the maximum possible relief.

Summary

The accurate and objective measurement of pain and its treatment is, therefore, complicated by numerous variables which are frequently not amenable to factual analysis. The patient's perceptions, hopes and fears, the variable nature of the disease, the influence of family, of culture and superstition, the strength of the influence of the doctor and the nurse, and the placebo effect all combine to make measurement imprecise. None the less, the attempt must be made if we are to make progress. As John Hunter said, 'Why argue gentlemen, why not try the experiment?'

References

Banning, A., Sjogren, P. and Henriksen, A. (1991) Treatment outcome in a multidisciplinary cancer pain clinic. *Pain*, **47**, 127–128.

Bookbinder, M., Coyle, N., Kiss, M. *et al.* (1996) Implementing national standards for cancer pain management: program model and evaluation. *J. Pain Sympt. Man.*, **12**(6), 334–347.

Bostrom, M. (1997) Summary of the Mayday Fund Survey: public attitudes about pain and analgesics. *J. Pain Sympt. Manage.*, **13**(3), 166–168.

Choiniere, M. and Amsel, R. (1996) A visual analogue thermometer for measuring pain intensity. *J. Pain Sympt. Manage.*, **11**(5), 299–311.

Cleeland, C.S., Gonin, R., Hatfield, A.K. *et al.* (1994) Pain and its treatment in outpatients with metastatic cancer. *New Engl. J. Med.*, **330**(9), 592–596.

De Conno, F., Caraceni, A., Gamba, A. (1994) Pain measurement in cancer patients: a comparison of six months. *Pain*, **57**(2), 161–166.

Grond, S., Zech, D., Diefenbac, C. *et al.* (1996) Assessment of cancer pain: a prospective evaluation in 2266 cancer patients referred to a pain service. *Pain*, **64**, 107–114.

McQuay, H., Carroll, D. and Moore, A. (1996) Variation in the placebo effect in randomised controlled trials of analgesics: all is as blind as it seems. *Pain*, **64**(2), 331–335.

Twycross, R.G. and Fairfield, S. (1982) Pain in far advanced cancer. *Pain*, **14**, 303–310.

Twycross, R.G., Harcourt, J. and Bergl, S. (1996) *Palliat. Med.*, **10**: 60.

Wall, P.D. (1992) The placebo effect: an unpopular topic. *Pain*, **51**, 1–3.

Ward, S.E., Goldberg, N., Miller-McCauley, V. *et al.* (1993) Patient related barriers to management of cancer pain. *Pain*, **52**, 319–324.

World Health Organization (1994) Revised method for relief of Cancer Pain and other symptoms management. WHO, Geneva.

The mechanisms of pain

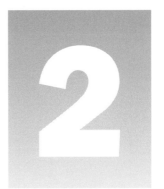

There exist in peripheral nerves groups of afferent nerve fibres which are devoted to the perception of pain. In the skin this appears to be their only function, whereas in the viscera it may well be that it is the frequency of firing of afferent impulses in general that gives the sensation of pain. These nerve fibres dedicated to pain perception are known as nociceptors. Stimuli picked up by these free nerve endings run either in the A delta sensory fibres, which are fast conducting, large diameter myelinated fibres, or in the C sensory fibres, which are slow, small and unmyelinated. Both types have their cell bodies in the dorsal root ganglia and both terminate in lamina II of the dorsal horn in the spinal cord, an area also known as the substantia gelatinosa. They then make a synapse with short neurones which synapse again very quickly, decussate across the mid-line, ascend in the anterolateral tracts of the white matter of the cord to the brainstem and eventually reach the thalamus. From there a further synapse carries them up to the level of the cerebral cortex. Here, for the first time, the pain messages impinge upon the conscious mind.

The synapses made between these neurones have chemical neurotransmitters to carry messages from one neurone to the next. These can either favour the pain messages or inhibit them. Such neurotransmitters include noradrenaline, substance P and vasoactive intestinal peptide (VIP). Some amino acids, such as glutamate, aspartate and homocysteine, are also known to act as neurotransmitters.

Transmission at these synapses can be blocked by several chemicals. Chief among them are the opioid peptides, which are grouped into three families, the endorphins, the dinorphins and encephalins, which all occur naturally in the body. Each has a specific opioid receptor, known as mu, kappa and delta, respectively. The mu receptors are by far the most important clinically because they are also the sites where exogenous opioids such as morphine and its many relatives have their activity.

In addition to opioid receptors other drugs, particularly ketamine, act as anti-nociceptor transmitters by disrupting the N-methyl-d aspartate (NMDA) mechanism. This is an excitatory amino acid receptor which is believed to sensitize the dorsal horn of the spinal cord to input from the peripheral sensory nerves. In addition to these methods of local transmission and inhibition, the body has its own inhibitory pathway running from the brainstem to the spinal cord. This blocks the transmission of pain messages in the spinal cord by inhibiting synaptic transmissions. The neurotransmitter for this mechanism is serotonin (5-hydroxytryptamine). A second descending inhibitory pathway running from the midbrain to the spinal cord has been recognized, for which the neurotransmitter is noradrenaline. Selective stimulation of these pathways produces analgesia in experimental animals. Tricyclic antidepressants such as amitriptyline block the re-uptake of serotonin and noradrenaline at the pre-synaptic level. They therefore enhance the inhibitory effect on nociception and it is believed that this is the reason for this group of drugs being effective in some cases of neuropathic pain.

This would seem a complex enough set-up, but the central nervous system has enormous capacity to modify, modulate and react to new situations. If a peripheral nerve is sectioned distal to the dorsal root ganglion, that ganglion itself will after 3–5 hours independently start firing a bombardment of afferent impulses (Wall, 1997). Also the denervated area will be twice as wide as the classical Sherrington map would indicate.

At the spinal level, other fibres, not normally given to carrying pain messages, can be pressed into service if the pain is constant or severe. Pain can therefore result from a light touch (allodynia) and can lead to hyperalgesia (feeling of intense pain from a slightly painful stimulus). Repeated stimuli transmitted into the spinal cord can also give rise to a vastly increased response within the spinal cord itself, so that neurones continue firing long after the stimulation has ended. This is known as 'wind up'. Finally, the cerebral cortex itself can become sensitized to pain, tuned in to the frequency at which pain is expected to occur. This undoubtedly causes the signal to be amplified at the highest levels when it arrives. This enormous adaptability, plasticity and subtlety of the central nervous system accounts for much of the variation in perception of pain seen in an individual person through the course of an illness. Add to that the enormous variation between one person and another in terms of sensitivity or stoicism, perception and reaction to painful stimuli, and the cultural, social and emotional variations that can occur and it is not surprising that pain is a complex subject.

Further analysis of the complexities of the basic neuroanatomy are beyond the scope of this book. Readers are referred to Twycross (1994) and of course to Wall and Melzack's *Textbook of Pain* (1984) and the *Oxford Textbook of Palliative Medicine* (Doyle *et al.* 1998).

References

Doyle, D., Hanks G.W.C. and MacDonald N. (1998) *Oxford Textbook of Palliative Medicine*, 2nd edn, Oxford University Press, Oxford.

Twycross, R. (1994) *Pain Relief in Advanced Cancer*, Churchill Livingstone, Edinburgh.

Wall P.D. (1997) *Pain*, 71, 1–3.

Wall P.D. and Melzack, R. (1984) *Textbook of Pain*, Churchill Livingstone, Edinburgh.

The opioid analgesic drugs

In 1986 the World Health Organization propounded its analgesic ladder, under the energetic chairmanship of Dr Jan Sternswjard. It has been recognized world wide as a valuable structure for treating cancer pain. The emphasis, as always in the treatment of disseminated cancer, is upon the treatment of the symptoms rather than upon the precise pathology. The three steps are as follows (see also Figure 10.5).

1. Patients with mild cancer-related pain should be treated with a non-opioid analgesic, combined with adjuvant drugs if there is an indication.
2. Patients with moderate pain and those failing to be pain free on step 1 should be treated with a weak opioid, often combined with a non-opioid and/or an adjuvant analgesic.
3. Patients with severe pain or who fail to be pain free on step 2 should receive a strong opioid, if necessary combined with a non-opioid and/or an adjuvant drug.

Over the past 10 years this analgesic ladder has been found to be a robust model of ideal treatment and has been widely used in developed and in developing countries wherever palliative care is practised. There have been several recent publications testing its validity. Zech *et al.* (1995) studied 2118 patients over a 10 year period in a pain service associated with palliative care. Eleven per cent of patients received step one treatment, 31% step two and 49% proceeded to step three. Eighty-two per cent received oral treatment, 9% were treated parenterally. Only 2% required spinal opioids and 6% other treatments. Twenty-six per cent received morphine. Co-analgesics such as antidepressants, anticonvulsants and corticosteroids were administered on 37% of treatment days. These authors reported a highly significant pain reduction within the first week of treatment ($P < 0.001$). Good pain relief was reported in 76%, satisfactory pain relief in 12% and inadequate pain relief in 12% of patients. In the final days of life 84% of patients rated pain as moderate or less, while 10% were unable to give a rating.

Zech *et al.* believe that because a full range of oncological adjuvant drug and non-drug treatment for pain were utilized the oral and parenteral morphine doses rarely exceeded 240 mg daily. Almost half of their patients required marked dose escalation, but they believed that this was because of the advance of progressive disease and therefore of increased pain. They did not believe drug tolerance to be a major clinical problem.

The same team reporting on a prospective study of 167 patients with head and neck cancer (Grond *et al.*, 1993) again found that the WHO ladder was effective in relieving pain. On 97% of a total of 8106 treatment days analgesics were administered. Severe pain was experienced only during 5% of the observation period. The most frequent symptoms observed were not pain but insomnia, dysphagia, anorexia, constipation and nausea. They concluded that the use of analgesic and adjuvant drugs given along WHO guidelines to treat pain was highly effective and relatively safe. Similar findings in head and neck cancer were reported by Talmi *et al.* (1997). They prospectively studied 62 consecutive patients with disseminated head and neck cancer. The visual acuity score (VAS) on admission was a mean of 4.7 (SD ± 2.0). A second mean VAS score 72 hours after the first was reduced to 1.9 (SD ± 1.1). This was statistically significant ($P < 0.001$). They found neuropathic pain to be present in 6 patients (12.5%), unlike other authors who have described neuropathic pain in 23–44% of head and neck cancers. Again, the WHO ladder was found to be valid and reliable.

Drugs for step 1

A study of controlled-release codeine compared with placebo showed that the active drug produced significantly lower pain scores and much less rescue analgesic consumption compared to placebo (2.2 ± 2.3 versus 4.6 ± 2.8 tablets per day, $P = 0.001$). The authors felt that controlled-release codeine given 12 hourly resulted in a significant reduction in pain intensity and that uninterrupted sleep and improved compliance were valuable benefits (Dhaliwal *et al.*, 1995).

In a meta-analysis of 30 randomized controlled trials Moore *et al.* (1997) located 31 trials of paracetamol versus placebo involving 2515 patients, 19 trials of paracetamol + codeine versus placebo with 1204 patients, and 13 trials of codeine versus paracetamol only where 874 patients were studied. The cut-off point applied was to identify the number of patients with at least 50% pain relief. To achieve this level, the number of patients needing to be treated (NNT) was on paracetamol 1 g 3.6, paracetamol 600 mg 5.0 and paracetamol 600 mg + codeine 60 mg 3.1. They therefore concluded that paracetamol is an effective analgesic and that adding codeine in a dose of 60 mg produces worthwhile additional pain relief.

These trials accord with clinical experience. Many patients with disseminated cancer never need more than paracetamol for much and sometimes for all their clinical course. Analgesia does not normally last longer than 4 hours and our practice is to give 1 g of paracetamol 4 hourly while the patient is awake, with the same dose to be taken through the night if the patient is awake and in pain. Aspirin is an equally effective step 1 drug, but in view of its known complications with dyspepsia and gastric haemorrhage it is considered not to be sufficiently more powerful than paracetamol to be used.

Drugs for step 2

The useful combination of paracetamol and codeine has already been mentioned. The main complication in using codeine in any form is its short action (maximum 4 hours) and its tendency to cause constipation, which means that the need to administer laxatives concurrently is considerable.

Dihydrocodeine is an analogue of codeine that is more powerful milligram for milligram but is less well absorbed, so parenteral medication is considerably stronger than oral. Thirty to sixty milligrams every 4–6 hours is usual, but many patients feel acutely confused and woozy on 60 mg and sometimes 30 mg every 2–3 hours is better tolerated. The slow-release preparation of this drug is available in many countries. Like codeine it can be constipating. Unlike codeine it must be given with caution in patients with impaired renal function.

Dextropropoxyphene is derived from methadone, and combined with paracetamol (marketed as Co-proxamol) is effective for moderate pain. One or two tablets 6 hourly will give good analgesia in many patients. The elderly may find this causes side-effects, particularly sedation and sometimes constipation. It had a bad press, owing to over-dosage, particularly combined with excessive alcohol, but currently it is generally believed that with sensible use it is safe and effective for many patients.

Tramadol is a newer analgesic acting centrally and having mild morphine-like effects. Its analgesic action is reversed by naloxone, as is that of morphine. It is usually given by mouth but can be given subcutaneously, intramuscularly, intravenously or rectally, and is normally well tolerated. Occasionally patients feel sick when taking it.

Grond *et al.* (1995) studied the racemic tramadol and compared it with its (+) and (−) enantiomers in patients recovering from gynaecological surgery in a double-blind trial. Of patients treated with (+) tramadol and the tramadol racemate, 12% and 15% respectively terminated the study because of inefficacy, but 53% of those receiving (−) tramadol stopped taking it because of inefficacy. Sixty-seven per cent of those patients taking

(+) tramadol were considered to be responders ($P = 0.061$) when compared with the racemate (48%) and (−) tramadol (38%) as judged by a five-point rating scale. When judged from the point of view of patient satisfaction with pain relief the figures were even more striking with 82%, 76% and 41% efficacy, respectively ($P = 0.001$). Nausea and vomiting were the most frequently reported non-serious side-effects and were most often seen with (+) tramadol. The authors concluded that taking into account both efficacy and safety, the racemate appeared to be superior to either of the enantiomers.

Moore and McQuay (1997) conducted a meta-analysis of 3453 post-operative patients in which oral tramadol was compared with placebo, codeine and combination analgesics in patients with moderate or severe pain after surgery or dental extraction. They found that tramadol and the other drugs all gave significantly more analgesia than placebo and that tramadol was equally effective with aspirin plus codeine and with paracetamol plus propoxyphene. The effects of tramadol were dose-related, for when comparing doses of 50, 100 and 150 mg the numbers needed to treat for 50% maximum relief were 7.1, 4.8 and 2.4, respectively. Adverse effects such as headache, nausea, vomiting and dizziness were similar in tramadol and the comparator drugs.

In clinical practice, subcutaneous tramadol is particularly useful in a syringe driver if the patient is for some reason unable to swallow or retain oral drugs and yet does not need strong opioids. It seems particularly unlikely to cause significant constipation. Nausea and vomiting are less than on morphine but can certainly be a problem in some patients. Haloperidol appears to be the specific antidote to this side-effect in a dose of 3–5 mg taken at night.

The strong opioids

It was Sir William Osler who said that morphine is God's own medicine. Certainly, morphine is the gold standard by which all other analgesic drugs are judged. It remains the bedrock for the treatment of severe pain due to cancer. In those countries where morphine is not easily available to aid the relief of suffering, the hands of the doctors are tied behind their backs. Their patients frequently are greatly distressed as a result. Indeed, the standard of specialist palliative care in a country may be measured by the amount of prescribed morphine consumed per head of the population.

In spite of this great boon to humanity, there has in the past been considerable reluctance to use morphine. In the 19th century, when extracts of opium became easily available, many literary people famously overdosed themselves upon it, often for long periods of time. As a result, morphine and its allied drugs fell under a cloud and eventually legislation was passed in Great Britain to control the prescribing and distribution of all the strong opioids. At the same time the general public became frightened of morphine. The phenomenon of 'opiophobia' is a complex one.

Many patients are worried about becoming drug addicts, of requiring more and more morphine to gain the requisite analgesia, of getting used to it so that it will not work when they really need it, and feel that a prescription for morphine is, if not a death sentence, at least an indication that the end is not far away. This was not helped by the attitude of many doctors, expressed by one in writing as 'I try to delay the administration of morphine for as long as I possibly can, and I try to ensure that the first dose of the drug is also the last.'

The preparation of opiate mixtures with other compounds such as chloroform water, alcohol, cocaine and chlorpromazine also obtained a bad name for opioids because the numerous side-effects of such cocktails were unpredictable and frequently very unpleasant.

It is now realized that there is no need for such mixtures. Straightforward morphine by mouth is normally adequate and effective if correctly prescribed. If swallowing is difficult, then subcutaneous or rectal routes can be employed.

Again, it was Dame Cicely Saunders who put the treatment of patients with morphine on to a rational and scientific footing. Her regimes at St Christopher's Hospice were the foundation of modern palliative medicine.

> It is a disgraceful episode in the history of medicine that doctors and scientists allowed themselves to join a mass hysteria which confused the tremendous benefits of narcotics for the patient in pain with the social abuse of the same compounds . . . The Brompton mixture is a pitiful example of unthinking medicine . . . a genuine cocktail of alcohol, cocaine, morphine . . . No wonder the population was suspicious when a group of doctors declared that 3 social evils (booze, snow and dope) were good for you. Wall, P.D. (1990) *Pain*, **43**, 267–268.

It was realized early that morphine, whether taken orally or by injection, would not last longer than 4 hours unless given in gross overdosage and that giving it every 4 hours by the clock was therefore essential if pain prevention was to be effective.

Indeed, pain prevention is the only standard of treatment that is acceptable. If the patient is allowed to experience pain and then has to take or ask for a dose of analgesic, he or she has to suffer pain until the dose is administered and becomes effective. When pain is inevitable, as it is with far advanced cancer in many cases, it is far preferable to accept that inevitability and to prevent rather than to treat it. This is not to say that some rescue medication for breakthrough pain should not also be prescribed in cases where the pain suddenly becomes stronger, or where another event occurs which means that a higher dose is needed. But the basic analgesia should always be by the clock.

Originally, morphine liquid was always used in oral preparations, but in recent years morphine tablets have become available which work as quickly and reliably as the liquids. Then we have slow-release morphine which lasts 12 hours (MST Napp or Oramorph SR Sanofi Winthrop). More recently, morphine preparations that last a full 24 hours (MXL Napp and Morcap Sanofi Winthrop) have been made available. Once the total daily dose of morphine has been titrated by 4 hourly doses against the pain experienced, then the total 24 hour requirement can be administered in a single once daily dose. This saves the patient's and the nurse's time, reduces the number of tablets that have to be taken, and avoids constant reminders for the patient that he or she is sick and requires medication.

The side-effects of morphine are mainly divided into the physiological and the toxic. Almost everyone when started on morphine, if they are naive to weak or strong opioids, will feel mildly sedated for 3–5 days. This does not mean that they are constantly asleep but rather that they will tend to nod off if nothing exciting or stimulating is happening, and that their normal drive and highest intellectual function is a little impaired. Usually this wears off, though in a few patients it persists.

Virtually everybody taking morphine will become constipated. This is not quite invariable because if patients have had a hemicolectomy in the past, their bowel function normally remains unaffected or only slightly harder. The vast majority, however, become obstinately constipated and the most distal masses of faeces become rock hard by long continued absorption of water. If laxatives are started, the result is either severe colic as the gut responds to stimulation to expel these rocks, or very frequently spurious diarrhoea, if softeners such as lactulose or docusate are given. The complaint of diarrhoea can then mean the prescription of drugs such as loperamide, while constipation giving colic often gets the patient more and more opiates, so aggravating the problem. One example that may be cited is that of a patient with metastatic carcinoma of lung who was admitted to a hospice with intractable abdominal pain not relieved by MST, which had been steadily increased to 160 mg b.d., with no laxatives. He was found to be severely constipated. Morphine was reduced and stopped, and after energetic measures to restore normal bowel function he was discharged home, pain free and on no analgesics at all.

The only safe precaution against opiate-induced constipation is to give both a stimulant and a softening laxative mixed together at the start of treatment. The hand that writes the prescription for morphine should be the hand that writes the prescription for a laxative on the same piece of paper on the same day. Usually co-danthramer or co-danthrusate is given and if constipation results despite this the dose is steadily increased or the prescription changed to strong co-danthrusate 5–10 ml at night. This is very much more effective but many patients dislike the vile taste and prefer large numbers of co-danthrusate capsules (Normax). Some patients, even without constipation, can develop quite severe colic as a result of taking co-danthramer preparations and in these cases it may be preferable to give a softener such as docusate or lactulose, and a small amount of senna. Senna should never be given in isolation.

The third common physiological side-effect of morphine is nausea, often coupled with protracted vomiting. This will occur in two-thirds of all patients who are naive to opioids when they first encounter morphine. It may be prevented in 95% of such patients by concurrent or, even better, pre-medication with haloperidol 3–5 mg at night. This powerful antiemetic works directly on the area postrema in the floor of the fourth ventricle of the brain. Here is situated the chemoreceptor trigger zone (CTZ) which is specific for morphine. It is rich in receptors, which pick up the presence of the drug in the cerebrospinal fluid and bloodsteam and through the dopamine mechanism activate the vomiting centre in the medulla. Haloperidol reliably blocks this central effect of morphine. Five per cent of patients will also require a prokinetic such as metoclopramide 10 mg t.d.s. because in these few subjects morphine also has a peripheral effect giving rise to gastric stasis.

The vomiting induced by morphine is characteristic. The patient constantly feels sick. Nothing relieves the patient, who will often sit for hours clutching the vomit bowl, convinced that any minute it will be required. Even when vomiting has occurred the patient feels no better; there are repeated small volumes ejected from the stomach (Figure 3.1) and even when it is completely empty the patient is often troubled by dry heaving and retching, which is most distressing. This contrasts sharply with the vomiting caused by gastric stasis such as is seen in pyloric obstruction or high intestinal obstruction in the duodenum or proximal jejunum. Here the vomiting is copious, almost without warning, consisting of several litres of gastric juice and food residues (Figure 3.2). Immediately afterwards the patient feels very much better, often hungry, can happily resume eating and drinking, and remains quite untroubled for several hours until another large-volume vomit occurs.

The toxic side-effects of morphine are quite different. These are seen when a patient is being over-treated with a strong opioid. In this situation the patient is not mildly sleepy or inattentive but will fall fast asleep and is almost unrousable. Often patients will fall asleep while the doctor is talking to them and I have known patients who fell asleep while they were actually

Figure 3.1
Vomiting due to opioids.
(Courtesy of Steve
Desmond.)

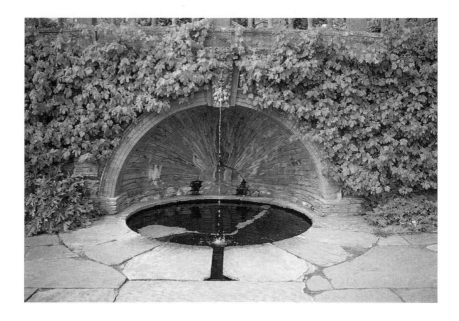

speaking to the doctor – suddenly the voice would falter and halt, the eyes would roll up and the eyelids droop, and the patient would be fast asleep. When awake, the patient frequently suffers from vivid visual hallucinations. Patients often conceal this because they think they are losing their minds,

Figure 3.2
Vomiting due to
obstruction of gastric
outflow. (Courtesy of Steve
Desmond.)

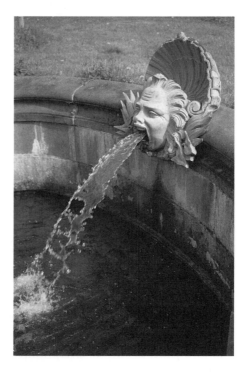

but if asked directly they will readily agree that they are seeing people, animals or insects jumping or crawling, sometimes in the front of their field of vision, sometimes around the periphery. Such patients also frequently display two characteristic physical signs. The pupils constrict down to tiny pin-point dots, which, if not present before morphine was started, strongly indicate overdosage. Also the limbs, particularly the hands and forearms, will display a characteristic intermittent myoclonic jerking. This frequently causes plates or teacups to be dropped and sometimes can be so violent that the contents fly over the patient's shoulder or into a visitor's face. These symptoms and signs indicate that the patient is on too high a dose of morphine, and that it must be reduced if the final toxic effect of respiratory depression is not to supervene.

Such toxic effects are not uncommon, because from first being reluctant to prescribe morphine, many doctors now are overenthusiastic, even pre-scribing it when the patient has no pain whatsoever, in the mistaken belief that if the patient has cancer he or she must need morphine. Little account is taken of the size of the patient or of his or her metabolic capabilities, so that the same dose is given to a 25 year old, 90 kg man, as to an 85 year old woman with carcinoma of the ovary and acute renal failure.

Morphine depends upon good kidney function for excretion of both the active drug and its two potent and metabolically active metabolites, morphine 6 gluconuride (M6G) and morphine 3 gluconuride (M3G), and it must therefore be given with great caution if there is a degree of renal failure present, and titrated very precisely to obtain the best possible effect with the minimum side-effects.

In a patient with renal failure and pain that is expected to be morphine-sensitive, it is wise to start with as little as 1 mg of morphine every hour and then titrate up according to the response of the pain and the size of the pupils. In the presence of renal failure, it takes a long time for the patient to excrete morphine and its metabolites. Even if treatment is stopped it can take 3 days before the toxic symptoms and the signs disappear (Tables 3.1 and 3.2). This principle can be shown by the first and second morphine equations:

$$M \rightarrow N\,V^2 \text{ (where M morphine and N V = nausea and vomiting)}$$
$$M + U + M3G + M6G \uparrow \rightarrow \uparrow N\,V^{10} \text{ (where U = uraemia)}$$

To avoid these side-effects other opioids have been extensively studied. Hydromorphone has become popular, particularly in North America, and is now available in the United Kingdom as palladone (Napp). This drug is seven times more powerful milligram for milligram than morphine, though this figure is based upon single-dose studies (Table 3.3). Dunbar *et al.* (1996) compared the two drugs in patient-controlled analgesia after bone marrow transplantation, when patients experienced severe oral mucositis. In

Table 3.1

Concentrations of morphine, M3G and M6G in a patient with renal failure given papaveretum

Time after opioid was stopped (h)	Respiratory depression	Morphine (nmol/l)	M3G[a] (nmol/l)	M6G[b] (nmol/l)
40	Yes	39	10220	2342
62	Yes	< 10	9230	2026
117	Yes	< 10	9720	1562
135	Yes	< 10	7670	1350
161	Yes	< 10	5040	1023
185	Yes	< 10	4940	872

[a] In this patient, plasma half-life of M3G = 136 h.
[b] In this patient, plasma half-life of M6G = 103 h.
Reprinted with permission from R.G. Twycross, *Pain Relief in Advanced Cancer*, Churchill Livingstone, 1994 (after Osborne *et al.*, 1986).

102 patients studied for up to 50 days (981 patient days) they considered the ratio of 3:1 to be more appropriate than 7:1. Further evidence is required to decide this important point. Lesser *et al.* (1996) studied hydromorphone in subcutaneous implants in animals and considered that the device gave safe and reproducible release of hydromorphone without any initial burst of drug release. They considered that this could provide a sustained subcutaneous infusion for patients, thereby improving pain control and compliance, and reducing concern about illicit utilization of opioids. However, it is not yet commercially available for patients.

Table 3.2

Oral morphine: influences on morphine and metabolite plasma concentrations

Factor	Effect
Age > 70 years Plasma creatinine > 150 mmol/l	M3G & M6G increased
Male	Morphine & M6G decreased
Ranitidine	Morphine increased
Elevated plasma creatinine + concurrent ranitidine	M6G increased
Elevated plasma creatine + concurrent tricycle antidepressants	MG3 increased

Reprinted with permission from R.G. Twycross, *Pain Relief in Advanced Cancer*, Churchill Livingstone, 1994 (after McQuay *et al.*, 1990).

	Dose conversion morphine (mg)	
Hydromorphone capsules (mg)		
1.3	10 ⎫	
2.6	20 ⎭	4-hourly
Hydromorphone SR capsules (mg)		
2	15 ⎫	
4	30 ⎪	
8	60 ⎬	12-hourly
16	120 ⎪	
24	180 ⎭	

Table 3.3
Hydromorphone

Dextromoramide is widely used in hospices when it is known that a treatment or dressing is bound to cause pain. It is claimed that this drug is rapidly absorbed from the buccal mucosa and therefore if 5–10 mg is given sublingually, when the tablet is completely dissolved it is possible to undertake the procedure under cover of an intense short burst of increased analgesia. However, Jones *et al.* (1996) studied the pharmacokinetics of 5 mg given sublingually and by slow intravenous injection to five volunteers. They found that the sublingual tablet was very variable in dissolving and the blood levels were much lower than those obtained by slow intravenous infusion. They therefore felt that dextromoramide could not be recommended for the indication that it is commonly given.

Faull *et al.* (1994) studied dipipanone elixir in three patients who were intolerant of morphine side-effects. They were able to obtain good pain relief with dipipanone powder made into an elixir in a dose of 5–15 mg 6 hourly. This was given without the cyclizine that is commonly compounded with this drug in the United Kingdom. No adverse effects upon cognition were observed. Maddocks *et al.* (1996) studied 13 patients who had been delirious on morphine and transferred them to subcutaneous oxycodone in a dose of between 15 and 250 mg per 24 hours. They observed lessened nausea and vomiting ($P < 0.05$) and also better mental state and pain relief. They point out, however, that rather less than 10% of the population are poor metabolizers of oxycodone because of a lack of the enzyme CYP2D6. This can be tested for by giving 30 mg of dextromethorphan, which is metabolized by this enzyme to dextrofan, which may be found in an 8-hour urine collection. Absence of dextrofan in the urine will therefore indicate that the patient would not tolerate oxycodone well.

Methadone has been the subject of several recent investigations because it has many attractions. It is very cheap, a powerful analgesic and is normally

Table 3.4

Properties of methadone compared to morphine

No active metabolite
Long half-life
Cumulation when given regularly
Longer duration of action
Faeces a major route of excretion
Renal failure does not alter pharmacodynamics
Nonlinear relationship between plasma concentration and analgesia
SC injection more likely to cause local reaction

Reprinted with permission from R.G. Twycross, *Pain Relief in Advanced Cancer*, Churchill Livingstone, 1994.

well tolerated (Table 3.4). Ripamonti, Zecca and Bruera (1997) reviewed this drug recently but found its use limited by its long and unpredictable half-life, the large variations between different individuals in handling it, the possibility of delayed toxicity, and the limited knowledge of how much and how often it should be given. Standard ratios with morphine were considered unreliable, particularly if patients had become tolerant to high doses. They therefore felt that methadone should not be given except in specialist units where very careful monitoring could be undertaken. Fainsinger, Schoeller and Bruera (1993) had come to similar conclusions. None the less, methadone can be of enormous help in particularly difficult situations. Thomas and Bruera (1995) described one patient with severe pain in the L5 vertebra who was on 'enormous doses of everything with no relief', for example hydromorphone 200 mg per hour. This patient was changed to methadone starting with 200 mg and increasing to 800 mg 6 hourly. Other drugs were tailed off and pain control remained perfect up to death. Rimmer and Trotman (1996) described nine patients who they believed had become insensitive to opioids. They were being treated with either 400–800 mg of morphine per day or 400–4000 mg of diamorphine per day and their pain was not controlled. Their treatment was converted to methadone in a ratio of 1:10 of the previous total daily dose of morphine or its equivalent, up to a maximum of 40 mg of methadone per dose. They were then titrated to either a 12 hourly or 8 hourly dosage. Six of the nine patients became stabilized after 3 to 11 days (median 4.5) on between 40 and 160 mg of methadone per day (median 90 mg). Three of these were fully relieved and two markedly improved, while in one there was only moderate improvement. Two died, of whom one had been totally relieved.

Treatment of one was discontinued after 5 days with no improvement. Only one patient was mildly drowsy.

Fentanyl

Fentanyl is a synthetic opioid which is very much more powerful than morphine, with a conversion ratio of 1:100. It is not well absorbed by mouth and until recently was used mainly by anaesthetists for post-operative pain. Given in subcutaneous boluses it is effective when the pain is short term and self-limiting, but this is not ideal for patients with cancer when the pain is inevitable and the analgesia therefore needs to be continuous. It can be given by continuous subcutaneous or intravenous infusion using a syringe driver, but recently a novel preparation giving fentanyl through the skin has been formulated as Durogesic (Janssen). Because fentanyl is very much more lipophilic than morphine it is readily absorbed through the transdermal route; it also crosses the blood–brain barrier more effectively to reach the central opioid receptors with ease. This is probably the reason for it being so much more powerful than morphine. In adequate doses fentanyl is very effective in relieving opioid-sensitive pains. Its main advantage lies in its relative freedom from side-effects (Figure 3.3).

In a series of 202 patients with cancer requiring strong opioid analgesia Ahmedzai and Brooks (1997) conducted a randomized open cross-over study comparing transdermal fentanyl with sustained-released oral morphine. Each patient received one treatment for 15 days followed immediately by the other for an equal period. Both treatments were equally effective in terms of pain control but fentanyl gave significantly less constipation ($P \leq 0.001$) and less daytime drowsiness ($P = 0.015$). However, sleep was shorter and more frequently disturbed than in patients with morphine. Of 136 patients who could express a preference, significantly more preferred fentanyl ($P = 0.037$), probably because of lessened side-effects. In clinical practice patients do indeed sometimes complain of wakefulness, particularly if they have become used to the sedative effects of continuous morphine. They also find that their highest intellectual functions work better on fentanyl.

In both the following cases the high-grade intelligence of one and the diminished cognitive function of the second clearly were impaired by morphine but preserved with equivalent doses of fentanyl, to the great pleasure of the patients and their relatives.

Grond *et al.* (1997) carried out a prospective study of 50 patients with advanced cancer of the gastrointestinal tract or head and neck requiring strong analgesia. The patients were allowed initially to titrate their own dose

Case report

A 72-year-old man with carcinoma of lung and chest-wall metastases required strong analgesia towards the close of his life. He was an academic whose aim was to remain in total mental control of his illness and his body to the end of life. On a non-steroidal anti-inflammatory drug (NSAID) plus morphine he was pain free, but found that his brain would not function as well as it normally did. He could not keep up intellectual discussions with his friends when they visited him and he greatly disliked this diminution in mental prowess. When changed to fentanyl his analgesia was equally effective but his brain regained full activity. He was able to do *The Times* crossword in his normal 8.5 minutes!

Case report

A 68-year-old man had carcinoma of prostate with bony metastases. Pain from these was controlled with an NSAID plus radiotherapy, but he then sustained an infarct in one parietal lobe of his brain. This left him mildly demented though fully active. He was intellectually impaired but could hold a simple conversation, feed himself and remained continent. As the cancer progressed he required stronger analgesia and when morphine was introduced, although it abolished the pain, he became aggressive, noisy, dirty and unco-operative. His wife, who cared for him devotedly, was greatly distressed by this change in his personality. His medication was changed from morphine to fentanyl and on the equivalent dose he remained pain free but regained his normal sunny disposition.

requirements of fentanyl delivered intravenously through a patient-controlled portable pump (demand dose 50 μg, lock-out time 5 minutes, hourly maximum dose 250 μg). On the second day of treatment the first transdermal patch was applied, with the delivery rate being calculated from the total patient administered dose of the first 24 hours. Intravenous fentanyl was also available on the second and third day, but thereafter oral or subcutaneous morphine was available as rescue medication. Adjuvant analgesics were also administered together with non-opioid analgesics as required. The patients were treated for 66 ± 101 days (range 3–535 days). The average daily delivery rate of fentanyl was 5.9 ± 4.1 mg. Initially the pain intensity, measured on a 101 point numeric analogue scale, was 45 ± 21. This decreased to 19 ± 15 during the phase of titration, and to 15 ± 11 during long-term treatment. Apart from three patients with moderate respiratory depression, severe side-effects were not observed. Compliance

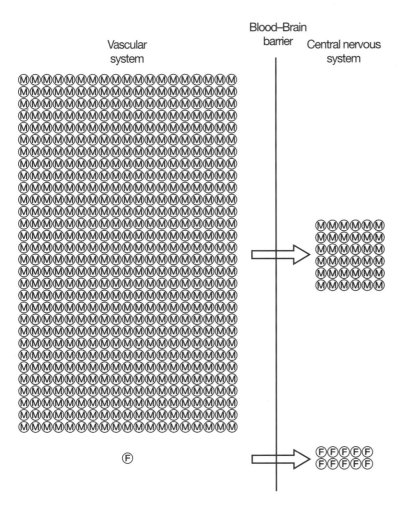

Figure 3.3
Distribution of equipotent doses of morphine and fentanyl in the vascular and central nervous systems based on animal data. Converting from oral or parenteral morphine to transdermal or parenteral fentanyl will result in a massive decrease in opioid molecules outside the CNS. This will result in less constipation and could, in physically dependent subjects, precipitate peripherally mediated withdrawal symptoms. Further, because opioids within the brain have an antiemetic effect (in contrast to opioids in the vascular system), it can be predicted that fentanyl will cause less nausea and vomiting than morphine. (Reprinted with permission from R.G. Tywcross, *Symptom Management in Advanced Cancer*, Radcliffe Medical Press, 1992).

and acceptance was good, and the authors commented that there was a marked reduction of both constipation and nausea. In three patients transdermal fentanyl failed because they required rapid escalation of doses which could not be achieved by the transdermal route.

The same team had already reported a multicentre study of 98 patients who had been transferred directly from oral morphine to transdermal fentanyl with a ratio of 100:1 daily (Donner *et al.*, 1996). The dosage of fentanyl was adjusted up or down according to the patients' needs and their VAS scores, together with the amount of liquid morphine required for rescue medication, were recorded. Analysis at the end of the study revealed a mean morphine/transdermal fentanyl ratio of 70:1 rather than the initially assumed 100:1. Pain relief on fentanyl and on morphine was identical, but constipation and laxative medication were significantly decreased during fentanyl therapy. Ninety-four point seven per cent of the patients chose to continue the transdermal fentanyl therapy at the end of the study. The authors recommend the initial conversion ratio of 100:1 as being safe and normally effective, though an increase in fentanyl may be required. Three of their patients developed a morphine-withdrawal syndrome during the first 24 hours of transdermal fentanyl therapy. This has become increasingly recognized as fentanyl has become more widely used. In such cases the patient becomes distressed and anxious, sweats profusely and feels acutely unwell. When recognized, this syndrome is easily and effectively treated by small rescue doses of morphine, decreasing in amount and frequency over 3–5 days. If the patient is pyrexial, absorption of fentanyl may be increased due to capillary vasodilation. This may also happen if mild respiratory depression causes CO_2 retention (Regnard: personal communication).

Care is needed in disposing of the used patches. They have already been seen in one house holding up the TV aerial, and in another replacing an elastoplast on a child's cut knee!

Opioid rotation

It sometimes happens that increasing the dosage of a strong opioid for severe pain produces proportionately less and less response in relief of symptoms. Rotating the treatment through different drugs is then well worth trying, provided that the pain is thought still to be opioid-sensitive. It is worth changing from morphine or diamorphine to methadone, hydromorphone or fentanyl. A retrospective survey of 80 patients undergoing 111 rotations showed that pain improved and cognitive function was less impaired in a significant number of patients, on less than equianalgesic doses (De Stoutz, Bruera and Suarez-Almazor (1995). In a review of opioid rotations, Fallon (1997) concluded that a switch could be helpful at times, but that avoiding toxic side-effects, such as confusion, and preventing dehydration and consequent biochemical upsets was fundamental. It was particularly important to ensure that fluid intake was sufficient to excrete morphine and its metabolites effectively – many patients do not drink enough.

Pethidine

Pethidine has no part to play in the treatment of chronic pain, for it is ineffective and toxic (Table 3.5).

Shorter duration of action
Ceiling effect because of toxic metabolite
Not antitussive
Less constipating
Less smooth muscle spasm (e.g. biliary tract, sphincter of Oddi)
More vomiting
Anticholinergic effects
Pupils not constricted
Metabolism → norpethidine; causes tremors, multifocal myoclonus, agitation, convulsions
Interactions with:

- phenobarbitone ⎱
- chlorpromazine ⎰ increase production of norpethidine
- monoamine oxidase inhibitors

Reprinted with permission from R.G. Twycross, *Pain Relief in Advanced Cancer*, Churchill Livingstone, 1994.

Table 3.5
Properties of pethidine compared to morphine

Naloxone

This drug is the specific antidote to morphine. It works in the mu-receptors as a morphine antagonist and is specific for patients who are in danger of dying due to morphine overdosage. In the palliative care setting this occurrence should be very rare, but it can happen that the patient either deliberately or accidentally takes a gross overdosage. It can happen also in a patient naive to opioids if they are acutely given too much of a strong opioid drug. A third situation can arise if a patient with severe pain, often taking large amounts of morphine or another strong opioid, is given an alternative analgesic procedure, e.g. amputation of a gangrenous limb or an epidural or intrathecal block which abolishes pain. In such situations the morphine dosage may be reduced to one-tenth or less of the previously required dose and this reduction must be rapidly achieved if the patient is not to suffer respiratory depression. If naloxone is required, it should be given intravenously in boluses of 0.4 mg in 10 ml saline. Long-acting opioids may require repeated doses, since naloxone has a short half-life in the body.

References

Ahmedzai, S. and Brooks, D. (1997) Transdermal fentanyl versus sustained-release oral morphine in cancer pain: preference, efficacy, and quality of life. *J. Pain Sympt. Manage.*, **13**, 254–261.

De Stoutz, N., Bruera, E. and Suarez-Almazor, M. (1995) Opioid rotation for toxicity reduction in terminal cancer patients. *J. Pain Sympt. Manage.*, **10**, 378–384.

Dhaliwal, H.S., Sloan, P., Arkinstall, W.W., *et al.* (1995) Randomized evaluation of controlled-release codeine and placebo in chronic cancer pain. *J. Pain Sympt. Manage.*, **10**, 612–623.

Donner, B., Zenz, M., Tryba, M. and Strumpf, M. (1996) Direct conversion from oral morphine to transdermal fentanyl: a multicenter study in patients with cancer pain. *Pain*, **64**, 527–534.

Dunbar, P.J., Chapman, C.R., Buckley, F.P. and Gavrin, J.R. (1996) Clinical analgesic equivalence for morphine and hydromorphone with prolonged PCA. *Pain*, **68**(2–3), 265–270.

Fainsinger, R., Schoeller, T. and Bruera, E. (1993) Methadone in the management of cancer pain: a review. *Pain*, **52**, 137–147.

Fallon, M. (1997) Opiod rotation: does it have a role? *Palliat. Med.*, **11**(3), 177–178.

Faull, C., MacKechnie, E., Riley, J. and Ahmedzai, S. (1994) Experience with dipipanone elixir in the management of cancer related pain. *Palliat. Med.*, **8**(1), 63–65.

Grond, S., Zech, D., Lynch, J. *et al.* (1993) Validation of World Health Organization guidelines for pain relief in head and neck. *Ann. Otol., Rhinol. Laryngol.*, **102**(5), 342–348.

Grond, S., Meuser, T., Zech, D. *et al.* (1995) Analgesic efficacy and safety of tramadol enantiomers in comparison with the racemate: a randomised, double-blind study with gynaecological patients using intravenous patient-controlled analgesia. *Pain*, **62**, 313–320.

Grond, S., Zech, D., Lehmann, K.A. *et al.* (1997) Transdermal fentanyl in the long-term treatment of cancer pain: a prospective study of 50 patients with advanced cancer of the gastrointestinal tract or the head and neck region. *Pain*, **69**, 191–198.

Jones, T.E., Morris, R.G., Saccoia, N.C. and Thorne, D. (1996) Dextromoramide pharmacokinetics following sublingual administration. *Palliat. Med.*, **10**, 313–317.

Lesser, G.J., Grossman, S.A., Leong, K.W. *et al.* (1996) In vitro and in vivo studies of subcutaneous hydromorphone implants designed for the treatment of cancer pain. *Pain*, **65** (2–3), 265–272.

Maddocks, I., Somogyi, A., Abbott, F. *et al.* (1996) Attenuation of morphine-induced delirium in palliative care by substitution with infusion of oxycodone. *J. Pain Sympt. Manage.*, **12**(3), 182–189.

Moore, R.A. and McQuay, H.J. (1997) Single-patient data meta-analysis of 3453 postoperative patients: oral tramadol versus placebo, codeine and combination analgesics. *Pain*, **69**, 287–294.

McQuay, H.J., Carroll, D., Faura, C.C. *et al.* (1990) Oral morphine in cancer pain : influences on morphine and metabolite concentration. *Clin. Pharmacal. Therap.*, **48**, 236–244.

Moore, R.A., Collins, S., Carroll, D. and McQuay, H. (1997) Paracetamol with and without codeine in acute pain – a qualitatative systematic review. *Pain*, **70**, 193–201.

Osborne, R.J., Joel, S.P. and Slevin, M.L. (1986) Morphine intoxication in renal failure: the role of morphine-6-glucuronide *Br. Med. J.*, **292**, 1548–1549.

Ripamonti, C., Zecca, E. and Bruera, E. (1997) An update on the clinical use of methadone for cancer pain. *Pain*, **70**, 109–115.

Rimmer, T. and Trotman, I. (1996) Methadone restores opioid sensitivity in cancer pain. *Palliat. Med.*, **10**(1), 58.

Talmi, Y.P., Waller, A., Bercovici, M. *et al.* (1997) Pain experienced by patients with terminal head and neck carcinoma. *Cancer*, **80**(6), 1117–1123.

Thomas, Z. and Bruera, E. (1995) Use of methadone in a highly tolerant patient receiving parenteral hydromorphone. *J. Pain Sympt. Manage.*, **10**, 315–317.

World Health Organization (1986) *Cancer Pain Relief*, WHO, Geneva.

Zech, D.F.J., Grond, S., Lynch, J. *et al.* (1995) Validation of World Health Organization guidelines for cancer pain relief: a 10-year prospective study. *Pain*, **63**, 65–76.

Bone pain

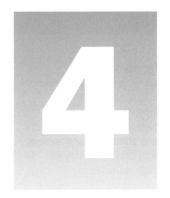

Cancers commonly metastasize to bone. Any malignant tumour may do so, but those that commonly present with bony metastases are tumours of lung, breast, kidney, prostate, multiple myeloma and thyroid. The metastases may be in a single bone or in many, and the pain arising from them may be the first intimation that the patient has cancer. Occasionally, a pathological fracture may be the presenting event.

The pain of a bony metastasis is typically a constant dull ache, accurately localized by the patient, often present at rest, but exacerbated by putting the bone under stress. Thus, a rib metastasis is made sharply more painful by coughing, laughing or taking a deep breath, while pain from metastases in the femur or tibia is greatly aggravated by standing or walking. Metastatic deposits in the pelvis are also exacerbated by weight bearing and may cause the legs to be unaccountably weak and unable to bear weight because of the instability of the origins of the thigh muscles (Figures 4.1 and 4.2). Metastases in the vertebrae are often confused with co-existing or presumed arthritis. The distinction can be difficult, but osteoarthritis of the spine selectively affects the middle cervical and lower lumbar facet joints. Cancer,

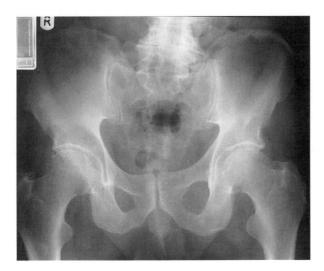

Figure 4.1
Carcinoma of prostate – normal pelvis.

Figure 4.2
Same patient as in Figure 4.1, 4 months later. Extensive bony metastases in left ischium and pubis, causing severe pain and instability of thigh muscles.

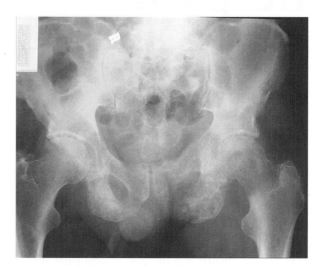

however, can metastasise to **any** vertebra. Osteoporosis can be confusing, particularly if only single vertebrae are affected, but the radiological appearances are different, for osteoarthritis produces a symmetrical collapse of vertebral bodies and it never destroys pedicles (Twycross, 1994; Table 4.1).

Vertebral metastases can be moderately or very painful, but may give surprisingly little in the way of symptoms until there is collapse of a vertebral body. The pain is then often very severe and localized to the vertebra in question, but it also gives rise either to a girdle pain, if an intercostal nerve is trapped, or to symptoms of spinal cord compression, if the fragments of bone impinge on the spinal canal. This is a palliative care emergency, for it may be possible to save the spinal cord and thereby prevent paraplegia if the cord can be saved (Figure 4.3). High-dose dexamethasone (16–24 mg daily) plus radiotherapy the same day that the diagnosis is made, and sometimes neurosurgical and orthopaedic stabilization of the spinal cord, should be considered. Speed of action is of the essence in this situation.

Impending fracture of a long bone similarly needs urgent if not emergency action. A series of 44 patients who had sustained a pathological fracture of femur were reviewed by McNamara and Sharma (1996). They estimated their Eastern Co-operative Oncology Group (ECOG) score in the week prior to sustaining the fracture. Twenty-three patients had an ECOG score of 3 or 4 and were evidently disabled. Ten of these were submitted to surgery but none managed to get home, surviving for a period of between 4 days and 5 months. The second group of 13 had an ECOG score of 2. All had surgery and six were able to return home. The remaining eight had an ECOG score of 0–1; all but one had surgery and all were rehabilitated at

A 40–60% change in bone density is necessary to detect changes on plain radiographs; pain can occur with less than this.

Plain radiographs are inadequate to evaluate where bone shadows overlap:
- base of skull
- C7, C8, T1 vertebrae
- sacrum.

Ordinary tomography of a vertebral body may distinguish between osteoporotic collapse and a metastasis.

Plain radiographs detect only 80% of osseous metastases.

Bone scans detect 95% of metastases.

Bone scans are sometimes negative in myeloma

Bone scan may show presence of a metastasis 3–6 months before plain radiograph. CT not often more helpful than isotope bone scan, but is procedure of choice for evaluation of retroperitoneal, paravertebral, pelvic and skull base areas.

It is sometimes necessary to proceed with treatment on the basis of clinical judgement alone.

Reprinted with permission from R.G. Twycross, *Pain Relief in Advanced Cancer*, Churchill Livingstone, 1994.

Table 4.1
Diagnostic radiology and cancer pain

home successfully. The 13 patients who were managed conservatively without surgery lived for between 2 days and 10 months, and none had problems with pain control. The authors concluded that the ECOG was a useful simple tool for assessing the likely outcome of pathological fracture, and suggested that for many patients whose previous state of health had been poor, surgery was contraindicated and did not lead to successful rehabilitation. Nor was surgery essential to secure adequate relief of pain.

If a femur or indeed any long bone is seen to contain a metastasis which occupies more than 50% of the width of the shaft, then the bone is going to fracture. The only question is when. Reactive treatment indicates that one leaves the patient alone until the fracture occurs and then attempts to stabilize the situation with the patient in great pain, shocked and sometimes in poor condition. Not infrequently this disaster shortens the patient's life dramatically. Proactive treatment, on the other hand, dictates that the fracture is stabilized by nailing or plating before the fracture occurs, when the patient is in good condition, the bone is in perfect alignment and the

Figure 4.3
Carcinoma of oesophagus with metastases in neck. MRI scan showing severe compression of spinal cord at L3–4. Immediate radiotherapy prevented quadriplegia, and greatly improved analgesia.

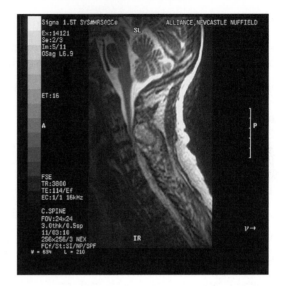

procedure is an elective one. Post-operative radiotherapy will then stabilize that metastasis and the patient is likely to live for both a longer and a happier term.

Case report

A 61-year-old woman with carcinoma of breast was being managed in a palliative care out-patients. She was happy, asymptomatic and enjoying her daily life over a period of several months. Suddenly, pain in her left femur became apparent, worsened rapidly and within 4 days her family doctor had obtained an X-ray, seen a large metastasis (Figures 4.4 and 4.5) and referred her urgently to an orthopaedic surgeon; within 5 days the femur was nailed and the patient made an uninterrupted recovery.

The sudden onset or rapid worsening of pain in a long bone therefore makes it mandatory to obtain urgent X-rays and to take action if a large metastasis is revealed (Figures 4.6–4.9).

The presentation of spinal cord compression in malignant disease was reviewed by Kramer (1992). He pointed out that spinal cord compression was not a terminal event, for 30% of patients survived for a year or more. Between 80 and 95% of all such patients presented with central localized back pain and vertebral tenderness. If compression of spinal nerve roots occurred, it was likely to be unilateral in the cervical and lumbar spine but bilateral in the thoracic spine. It caused the patient nearly always to need to

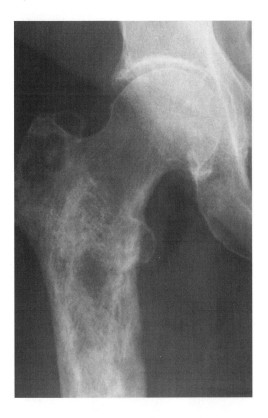

Figure 4.4
Metastases from
carcinoma of breast. See
case report on page 40.

sleep and sit upright because the pain was greatly exacerbated by lying flat. Cord compression, on the other hand, produced less sharp, more diffuse pain and often a cold unpleasant sensation. Both root compression and cord compression were made worse by coughing, sneezing, straining, straight leg raising or flexion of the neck, and the pain could precede the onset of physical signs by a median of 6.7 weeks, with the range being from 5 days to 2 years. The prognosis after treatment with high-dose steroids, radiotherapy, and surgery if radiotherapy failed was in general that the pre-treatment function was preserved but that there was little chance of improvement beyond that. Janjan (1996) confirmed that pain made worse on recumbancy and relieved by sitting up was present in 95% of patients and could occur days or months before neurological dysfunction could be detected. He also found that after radiotherapy the level of pre-treatment function was maintained at 3 years in 90% of survivors (Figures 4.10 and 4.11).

Treatment of bone pain

Opioids are of limited use in relieving the pain of bony metastases. Sometimes paracetamol or a moderate opioid such as co-proxamol or co-

Figure 4.5
Metastases from carcinoma of breast. See case report on page 40.

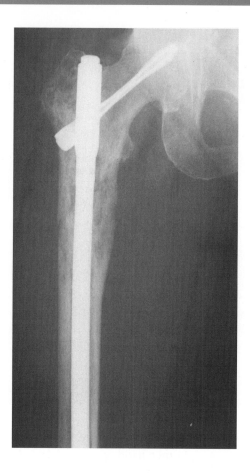

codamol are sufficient, but the bedrock of treatment remains the non-steroidal anti-inflammatory drugs (NSAIDs). These are specific for the bony pain that is experienced. Levick *et al.* (1988) carried out a multi-centre double-blind trial of naproxen in doses of 550 mg 8 hourly or 550 mg initially, followed by 275 mg 8 hourly. The patients evaluated their pain on a scale of 0–99. Pain scores were decreased by approximately one-third in each treatment group and among those patients who did respond to the drug, pain relief was significantly higher in the high-dose than the low-dose regime. Pace (1995) reviewed the use of NSAIDs in cancer, comparing their efficacy, their relative adverse effects and their tolerability. While agreeing with the useful role of NSAIDs in clinical practice for cancer pain generally and for bone pain in particular, an exhaustive search of the literature failed to find any randomized controlled trial of sufficient power to provide conclusive evidence, other than that of Levick *et al.* (1988). A large, well-designed trial of NSAIDs in bone pain is badly needed. Pace also reviewed the evidence for NSAIDs acting centrally, perhaps by modulating the wind-up phenomenon in the spinal cord, and raised the interesting possibility

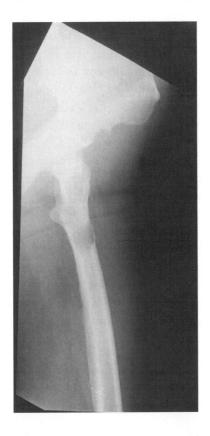

Figure 4.6
Fibrous histiocytic sarcoma of maxilla. Metastases in upper quarter of femoral shaft.

that in future NSAIDs designed to act in the central nervous system, perhaps by intrathecal injection, would be of value. Other authors differ in their belief in the power of NSAIDs to relieve bone pain. Regnard and Tempest (1998) and Twycross (1992) dismiss this group of drugs as being of little long-term help, but Kaye (1994) claims that NSAIDs will control bone pain in 80% of cases within a few days, with 60% of cases responding to any NSAID and 20% more on changing the NSAID. None of these authors produced conclusive evidence based on formal trials to support their beliefs.

The new NSAID ketorolac has attracted considerable interest because it appears to have a more specifically analgesic rather than anti-inflammatory role. Blackwell *et al.* (1993) described seven patients with bone pain treated with subcutaneous ketorolac in a dose of 30–60 mg per 24 hours plus misoprostol orally for between 8 and 31 days. The indications for this were either unresponsiveness or side-effects to opioids. All seven became pain free, four needed no opioid and the other three needed substantially less within a 29–60% reduction in total opioid dosage. They observed no side-effects and particularly no gastrointestinal bleeding. Middleton, Lyle and Berger (1996) gave ketorolac by continuous intravenous infusion in a dose of 240 mg daily over 90 days to a patient with intractable pain from metastatic carcinoma of the oesophagus with an excellent response. At one point the patient suffered a perforation of the oesophagus in an area where previous irradiation had been applied. The ketorolac was discontinued, but the pain became so intense that the drug had to be resumed and again give extremely good results. Duncan, Hardy and Davis (1995) gave 10 patients ketorolac subcutaneously for between 3 and 22 days in a dosage of 55–150 mg per day. The indications were inadequate analgesia with opiates ± NSAIDs. Five patients needed less opiate, four needed more and in one there was no change.

The main disadvantage of all the NSAIDs is the development of gastrointestinal complications, particularly dyspepsia and bleeding. Henry *et al.*[?] (1996) conducted a meta-analysis of this group of drugs. On the whole ibuprofen was associated with the lowest relative risk, but this was probably due to the low doses of the drug commonly used in clinical practice. In high doses, ibuprofen was associated with a similar risk to other NSAIDs. The next lowest risk drug was diclofenac. Indomethacin, naproxen, sulindac and

Figure 4.7
Same patient as in Figure 4.6. Prophylactic nailing of femur followed by palliative radiotherapy.

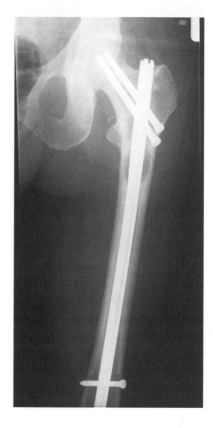

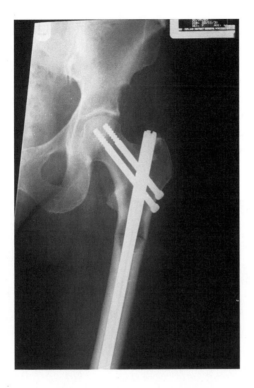

Figure 4.8
Same patient as in Figures 4.6 and 4.7. Transverse fracture of femur in spite of nailing and radiotherapy.

aspirin occupied intermediate positions. The highest risk drugs were asapromazone, tolmetin, ketoprofen and piroxicam.

These complications of NSAIDs may be reduced, but not abolished, by the concomitant administration of misoprostol. Problems arise when the patient has a past history of either definite gastric or duodenal ulceration or previous haemorrhage, either from an ulcer or from previous administration

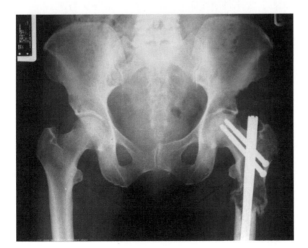

Figure 4.9
Same patient as in Figures 4.6, 4.7 and 4.8. Complete destructure of upper end of femur, including greater trochanter, and erosion of anterior edge of ilium by tumour.

of an NSAID. In all such situations the risk is markedly increased and the possible benefit has to be weighed against the real risk of a recurrence. The newer Cox-2 NSAIDs may be preferable here. Problems also arise if the patient is concurrently on an anticoagulant such as warfarin for co-existing deep vein thrombosis or previous heart surgery. Our practice if an NSAID is definitely required is to stop the anticoagulant for 24 hours, start the NSAID drug and then resume the anticoagulant at 50% of the dose and recalibrate the INR level.

Figures 4.10 and 4.11
MRI scans showing compression of cord due to collapse of T12. The patient's only symptom was of pain in the perineum and coccyx which resisted diagnosis and treatment until this distant cause became apparent. Radiotherapy to T12 produced rapid resolution of the pain.

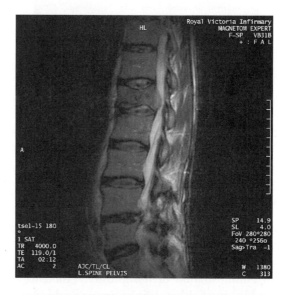

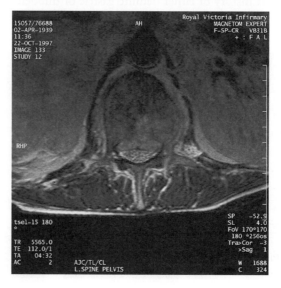

The other mainstay of the treatment of painful bony metastases is radiotherapy. This may be given as a single or several fractionated doses, according to site and the preference of the radiotherapist concerned. Needham, Mithal and Hoskin (1994) reviewed 97 patients who had radiotherapy at the Royal London Hospital for painful bony metastases. There was no departmental policy for how treatment was administered. Forty-one per cent of treated sites received a single fraction. There was particular reluctance to treat the cervical spine with single doses of irradiation. Seventy-nine per cent of metastases at this site received more than five fractions. This was also the case in metastases in the pelvis and hips, with 66% receiving more than five exposures. On the other hand, 95% of patients with rib metastases received only a single dose, and 54% of patients with long bone sites received single-dose treatment. No relationship was seen between response rates and the degree of fractionation or total dose. The overall response rate in this series for the three major groups of tumour were: prostate 84%, breast 87% and lung 63%. Hoskin (1995) reviewed the results of hemi-body irradiation, a technique that involves the use of a large external beam mega-voltage for widely scattered metastases, in either the upper or the lower half of the body. These treatments can be given consecutively provided there is a gap of 4–6 weeks between treatments to allow the bone marrow to recover. Increased gastrointestinal symptoms of nausea, vomiting and diarrhoea are reported from lower hemi-body irradiation, and nausea and occasional pneumonitis can complicate upper hemibody irradiation. Pre-medication with an antiemetic, steroids and intravenous hydration in hospital is recommended. Alternatively, the administration of radioactive strontium (^{89}Sr) can be used. The body handles strontium in the same way as calcium and it is therefore deposited in those bony sites where metabolism is most active. This delivers the radiation directly to every metastatic spot in the bony skeleton. An acute flare of pain for several days after radioactive strontium means that analgesia needs to be doubled or tripled in many cases. The other disadvantage of radioactive strontium is the high cost; on the other hand, the treatment can be taken to the bedside of a patient in pain rather than having to transport the patient to a radiotherapy centre.

Recent work has suggested that the bisphosphonate group of drugs, already widely used for the treatment of malignant hypercalcaemia, may relieve bone pain and prevent pathological fractures. These drugs act by inhibiting the osteoclast cells which actively resorb bone under the influence of local malignant cells. Robertson, Reed and Ralston (1995) undertook a double-blind randomized controlled trial of oral clodronate on metastatic bone pain. Fifty-five patients with progressive bony metastases received clodronate 1.6 g per day or a placebo. Pain measured by a visual analogue score decreased in the treated group but increased in the placebo group (P = 0.03) The use of analgesics increased with the progression of the disease in both groups. An equal number of patients in each group withdrew because of difficulty in swallowing the large capsules.

In a review of the management of bony metastases Mercadante (1997) quoted several trials where oral clodronate or intravenous pamidronate appeared to give a gradual but persistent reduction of bone pain. There was also some evidence that skeletal complications such as pathological fracture were diminished in advanced multiple myeloma and in breast cancer. On the other hand, another study on prostate cancer showed no evidence of improved pain control with oral clodronate (Hughes, Wilcock and Corcoran, 1997).

Other evidence of bisphosphonates being effective as analgesics, and as preventors of pathological fractions, was presented by Scott-Ernst *et al.* (1997), who conducted a double-blind cross-over study of clodronate 600 or 1500 mg versus placebo in 60 patients with metastatic bone disease and pain. There was no difference between the two doses, but 57% of patients ($P < 0.0021$) and 65% of investigators ($P < 0.0001$) preferred clodronate to placebo.

A particular problem arises with incident pain due to bony metastases. In this situation the patient is comfortable at rest but is in severe pain when active or passive movement is attempted. Relief of this by drugs is extremely difficult for to have the patient totally pain free, for instance when walking, means that at rest he or she will be on far too great a dose of analgesics. Often physical methods, such as splinting of the affected bone, is preferable to an increased drug load.

Case report

A man of 61 with primary carcinoma of lung was found to have a single metastatic deposit at the lower end of his left femur. He was given radiotherapy and an NSAID for pain but the tumour steadily increased in size and increasing amounts of morphine did nothing to relieve his pain on weight bearing. At rest he was completely comfortable. The tumour steadily expanded into the knee joint, across the joint space and into the upper tibia (Figure 4.12). An ischial bearing caliper was constructed which stabilized the limb and made him able to transfer and walk short distances in comfort. Orthopaedic intervention was considered but ruled out initially because of the advanced stage of the disease process. Amputation of the leg was considered but rejected. Eventually, the patient was asked by his wife to change a light bulb. He took off the caliper, climbed on to a table, received an electric shock from the fitting, and was thrown on to the floor, breaking the leg. Extensive orthopaedic surgery therefore became inevitable. Therefore the knee had to be stabilized using a high cast brace (Figure 4.13). This made the leg very much more

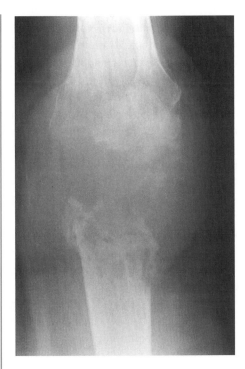

← Figure 4.12
Metastases from carcinoma
of lung in knee joint.

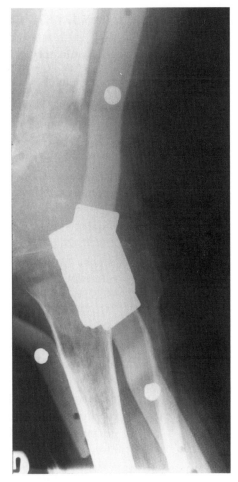

Figure 4.13 ▶
Immobilization in a brace.
See case report on page 48.

comfortable and stabilized the knee joint. The patient survived another 4 months and in spite of developing a Pancoast syndrome, which was treated with radiotherapy, and metastases in his adrenal glands, he remained well until developing a terminal bronchopneumonia and dying peacefully in his own home.

References

Blackwell, N., Bangham, L., Hughes, M. *et al.* (1993) Subcutaneous ketorolac – a new development in pain control. *Palliat. Med.*, 7, 19–25.

Duncan, A.R., Hardy, J.R. and Davis, C.L. (1995) Subcutaneous ketorolac. *Palliat. Med.*, **9**(1), 77–78.

Henry, D., L.-Y. Lim, L., Rodriguez L.A.G., *et al.* (1996) Variability in risk of gastrointestinal complications with individual non-steroidal anti-inflammatory drugs: results of a collaborative meta-analysis. *Br. Med. J.*, **312**, 1563–1566.

Hoskin, P.J. (1995) Radiotherapy for bone pain. *Pain*, **63**, 137–139.

Hughes, A., Wilcock, A. and Corcoran, R. (1997) Ketorolac: continuous subcutaneous infusion for cancer pain. *J. Pain Sympt. Manage.*, **13**(6), 315–316.

Janjan, N.A. (1996) Radiotherapeutic management of spinal metastases. *J. Pain Sympt. Manage.*, **11**(1), 47–56.

Kaye, P. (1994) *A to Z of Hospice and Palliative Medicine*, EPL Publications, Northampton.

Kramer, J.A. (1992) Spinal cord compression in malignancy. *Palliat. Med.* **6**(3), 202–211.

Levick, S., Jacobs C., Loukas, D.F. *et al.* (1988) Naproxen sodium in treatment of bone pain due to metastatic cancer. *Pain*, **35**, 253–258.

McNamara, P. and Sharma, K. (1996) Fractures in the palliative setting. *Palliat. Med.*, **10**, 59.

Mercadante, S. (1997) Malignant bone pain: pathophysiology and treatment. *Pain*, **69**, 1–18.

Middleton, R.K., Lyle, J.A. and Berger, D.L. (1996) Ketorolac continuous infusion: a case report and review of the literature. *J. Pain Sympt. Manage.*, **12**(3), 190–194.

Needham, P.R., Mithal, N.P. and Hoskin, P.J. (1994) Radiotherapy for bone pain. *Roy. Soc. Med.*, **87**, 503–505.

Pace, V. (1995) Use of non-steroidal anti-inflammatory drugs in cancer. *Palliat. Med.*, **9**(4), 273–286.

Regnard, C.F.B. and Tempest, S. (1998) *A Guide to Symptom Relief in Advanced Disease*, Hochland & Hochland.

Robertson, A.G., Reed, N.S. and Ralston, S.H. (1995) Pain relief into practice: rhetoric without reform (editorial). *J. Clin. Oncol.*, **13**(9), 2149–2151.

Scott-Ernst, D., Brasher, P, Hagen, N. *et al.* (1997) A randomised controlled trial of intravenous clodronate in patients with metastatic bone disease and pain. *J. Pain Sympt. Manage.*, **13**, 319–326.

Twycross, R.G. (1992) *Symptom Management in Advanced Cancer*, Radcliffe Medical Press, London and New York.

Twycross, R.G. (1994) *Pain Relief in Advanced Cancer*, Churchill Livingstone, Edinburgh.

Pain in bladder and bowel

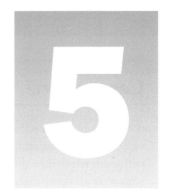

The essential feature of pain in hollow viscera such as the bladder and bowel is its intermittent colicky nature. When smooth muscle in the wall of the organ is stretched it responds by intermittent contractions which at first are imperceptible. Everybody's small and large intestine operate continuously with rhythmic peristaltic contractions which are not normally felt. Only when the organ is full and demanding evacuation do the contractions become strong enough to impinge on the conscious mind. Normally, in all of us, these result in easy micturition or defaecation and the contractions at once subside. If, however, normal emptying is impossible, the contractions become more and more insistent and increasingly painful. The bladder may be filled by a tumour or blood clot or the urethra occluded by a stone, clot or blocked catheter. Similarly, the small or large intestine can be blocked by a tumour either within the lumen or within the wall of the intestine, or by external compression from tumour masses, by adhesions or by interference with the normal sympathetic nervous system due to a tumour invading the mesentery. Blockage with rock-hard faeces owing to obstinate constipation can frequently mimic intestinal obstruction very closely.

Another type of bladder pain results from invasion of the base of the bladder by a metastatic tumour or primary prostatic cancer growing upwards. This typically produces terminal dysuria when, as the bladder contracts down at the end of micturition, the bladder base is moved and causes pain. This can be an early and often unrecognized symptom of pelvic cancer. Typically the pain is felt deep in the perineum and often referred to the glans penis.

Whenever possible, treatment is aimed at removing the cause of the obstruction. Cystoscopy can remove a blood clot and often reduce tumour bulk. External-beam radiotherapy can also be used to reduce the size of tumour masses within the bladder. Wherever possible, intestinal obstruction is treated by surgical resection or bypass of the lesion, but in patients presenting to palliative care units very few such subjects are found. Many have already been correctly dealt with by the surgical teams. Most others have either multiple sites of blockage or are in a poor state of general health

Case report

A 41-year-old man self-medicated himself for 2 years for haemorrhoids before his adenocarcinoma of rectum was discovered and resected. He was then well for 2 years but developed pain in the perineum referred to the penis at the end of micturition. Physical examination, cystoscopy and CT scan were all completely normal and it was several months before a metastatic tumour in the deep pelvic tissues eroding into the base of the bladder could be visualized on repeat scanning.

so that surgery is not feasible, or technically no bypass procedure is possible.

Traditionally such patients with intestinal obstruction were treated with intravenous fluids and nasogastric aspiration. This is easy to start in hospital, but if the patient is otherwise active and relatively well it is difficult to continue over a period that may last for many weeks. Therefore Dr Mary Baines and her colleagues at St Christopher's Hospice instituted the management methods that have now become standard in many units throughout the world. This involves the administration of continuous subcutaneous analgesia and antiemetics by syringe driver with the patient being allowed a free diet of liquids and whatever food he or she can take. The drugs typically used are hyoscine butylbromide (Buscopan) in a dose of 80–160 mg per 24 hours for pain; the usual antiemetic is cyclizine 150 mg per 24 hours. Sometimes diamorphine is required also in the syringe driver if pain is not controlled by Buscopan alone. With this regimen pain is abolished, nausea is normally well controlled and the patient will tolerate one or two vomits per day provided his or her quality of life is otherwise good (Baines, 1998). This is a regimen that can be started in hospital or in a hospice and then continued at home, where the patient can live as normal a life as possible for weeks or even months.

The vast majority of patients require no more, but some, particularly those with a high obstruction in the small intestine, have such copious vomiting that other methods are required. Recently the introduction of octreotide has greatly improved the control of symptoms in these patients. Octreotide is a synthetic drug closely related to the natural hormone somatostatin but with a half-life of 12 hours rather than 4 minutes. It works by inhibiting the secretion of gastric and intestinal juices and by promoting absorption of intestinal contents. The volume available to vomit is therefore markedly reduced. Dramatic improvements can often be obtained even in patients who have been vomiting for weeks or months. The dose used is 150–1200 µg per 24 hours by continuous subcutaneous infusion. Twice daily subcutaneous injections can be used, but they are painful. Riley and

Fallon (1994) reported a series of 35 cases of intestinal obstruction treated with octreotide which had been resistant to symptomatic relief with the usual St Christopher's regimen. The vast majority had their vomiting brought under rapid and complete control, and this persisted for the rest of their lives. Mercadante (1995) has recently reviewed the management of bowel obstruction in 25 patients over 4 years, and similarly found octreotide to be impressively successful.

For bladder pain, if the cause cannot be relieved, it is worth considering diversion of the urinary flow. A urethral catheter, suprapubic catheter or bilateral nephrostomies are all worth considering if the patient's distress is caused by the need to micturate. If, however, the pain is due to the continued presence of a solid object, such as tumour which cannot be passed and which is resistant to palliative radiotherapy or chemotherapy, then pharmacological measures are required. The pain is mainly caused by contraction of the detrusor muscle in the dome of the bladder. This is mediated by cholinergic fibres and therefore an anticholinergic drug is employed. Propantheline was widely used but the drug of choice now is oxybutynin (Ditropan). In a dose of 2.5–10 mg 8 hourly this markedly inhibits bladder contraction. Its main side-effect is a dry mouth and paralysis of visual accommodation. If it is insufficient alone to obtain comfort, opiates should be added in adequate amount to obtain pain relief.

References

Baines, M. (1998) The pathophysiology and management of malignant intestinal obstruction, in *Oxford Textbook of Palliative Medicine* (eds D. Doyle, G.W.C Hanks, and N. MacDonald), pp. 526–534. Oxford University Press, Oxford.

Mercadante, S. (1995) Bowel obstruction in home-care cancer patients: 4 years experience. *Supportive Care in Cancer*, **3**(3), 190–193.

Riley, J. and Fallon, M.T. (1994) Octreotide in terminal malignant obstruction of the gastrointestinal tract. *Euro. J. Palliative Care*, **1**, 23–25.

Nerve blocks

It is rare for patients with cancer to require nerve blocks but in those few patients whose pain problems are overwhelming a nerve block can be dramatically effective. The main indications for such an intervention are ineffective or insufficient pain relief with oral, subcutaneous or intravenous drugs. This situation can occur when the patient has either overwhelming pain or a mixed nociceptive and neuropathic pain complex, or when side-effects are intolerable and unmanageable. Such situations used to be managed by neurolytic techniques, i.e. surgical ablation of peripheral nerves by injection with alcohol or phenol. Such techniques are now rarely used because application of opioids and local anaesthetics, either in the epidural space or intrathecally, have proved to be far superior, easily maintained for long periods and do not involve destruction of tissues. Van Dongen, Crul and De Bock (1993) retrospectively reviewed 51 patients who were treated by continuous intrathecal morphine through a tunnelled percutaneous catheter. Seventeen of these also received bupivacaine together with morphine. Pain relief was improved in 10 and moderately improved in a further four patients. In the three who did not benefit there were clinical signs of severe mental depression. A gradual dose increment was observed in all patients and no serious complications were noted. Two patients eventually underwent percutaneous cervical cordotomy because they had persistent unilateral pain which could not be abolished by intrathecal treatment.

Krames (1993) reviewed intraspinal opioids and local anaesthetics for the relief of intractable pain. In a review of the literature he concluded that this was a good therapeutic alternative in those relatively few patients whose pain could not be controlled but that prospective blind controlled studies were required. He also quoted evidence in the literature of potential neural toxicity in rats of local anaesthetic agents used chronically.

Van Dongen, Van and Crul (1997) described five patients in whom intrathecal administration of morphine and bupivacaine was shortly followed by symptoms of compression of the spinal cord or cauda equina, confirmed radiographically. They suggested that new neurological symptoms presenting in this way may therefore be an early indicator of space-occupying lesions within the spinal canal.

Ten patients with severe cancer-related pain were studied in a randomized double-blind cross-over study comparing epidural and subcutaneous morphine (Kalso *et al.*, 1996). The patients titrated themselves until pain free over 48 hours using a patient-controlled analgesia system. The median daily doses were 372 mg for subcutaneous and 106 mg for epidural morphine. The two modes of administration were comparable in both effectiveness and acceptability. Both provided better pain relief with less adverse effects compared with the oral morphine given before the study.

In an analysis of patients receiving intrathecal or epidural analgesia in their hospice, Makin and Regnard (1994) found that the intrathecal route gave better analgesia, with less risk of the line being dislodged and no greater risk of infection or hypotension. Most hospices now prefer the intrathecal route to epidural blocks. In a one-year prospective study of 43 patients, Ellershaw *et al.* (1996) concluded that neural block (epidural, paraverterbrae or lumbar psoas) was an essential component of specialist palliative care.

Local nerve blocks are, however, sometimes used in specific instances. For severe pain from pancreatic cancer the best treatment is sometimes blockade of the coeliac plexus. This can relieve a pain that is notoriously difficult. Indeed, some surgeons now undertake coeliac plexus block at open operation when pancreatic cancer is found. More usually, however, the task is given to anaesthetists who use alcohol or phenol to destroy the plexus. Mercadante (1993) reported 20 such patients, 10 of whom were treated conservatively while the other 10 underwent coeliac plexus blocks. Those patients who were treated in the latter way achieved a reduction in opioid consumption compared with those receiving only oral analgesics. There was an equal reduction in VAS pain scores, though side-effects were a greater problem in the patients treated without the nerve block. De Conno *et al.* (1993) described a patient who developed paraplegia following a coeliac plexus block and found four other cases in the literature. An acute myelopathy was believed to have caused this complication.

Other nerve blocks are sometimes used, particularly chemical attack on the lumbar or cervical sympathetic chain for intractable pain in a leg or an arm. In skilled hands it can be very effective. This is particularly so in patients with Pancoast's syndrome, when the arm is not only painful but also wasted, cold and numb. Pelvic pain from cancer has been treated by neurolytic block of the superior hypogastric plexus (de Leon-Casasola, Kent and Lema 1993), who described 26 patients with incapacitating pelvic pain unrelieved by oral opioids and/or distressed by side-effects. They performed bilateral percutaneous neurolytic block with 10% phenol of the hypogastric plexus. The VAS pain score of all patients was 10/10 before treatment and 15 patients (69%) had satisfactory pain relief after one block and three others after a second block. The remaining eight patients (31%) had only moderate pain control and they were therefore treated with epidural bupivacaine and morphine with good results. Both groups were found to have significant reductions in oral opioid therapy. No complications were reported and the authors concluded that the technique was effective and well accepted by their patients.

Occasionally percutaneous cervical cordotomy is employed for unilateral pain. This technique is used to interrupt the lateral spinothalamic tract in the cervical spinal cord. Stuart and Cramond (1993) described 273 patients treated in this way. They claimed satisfactory pain relief in 89% of patients with a mortality of 3.3%. Long-term survivors over 8 and 5 years remained free of original pain. The authors concluded that the method was valuable for treatment of cancer pain in selected patients where the disease was unilateral, particularly in 114 patients who had primary lung cancer or mesothelioma. Bilateral cervical cordotomy is not possible because respiratory failure is a very great hazard.

With all such techniques it is essential to have the assistance of an anaesthetist (or in the case of cervical cordotomy a neurosurgeon) who is both skilled in the technique and readily available. Not infrequently the initial procedure even though successful requires a great deal of post-operative advice and further intervention. Therefore a good 'after sales service' is needed if the clinician is to avoid being placed in a very difficult position. There is no place for the doctor who likes to try his or her hand at the occasional nerve block, nor for one who undertakes the procedure but who is thereafter unavailable or disinterested in the clinical outcome.

References

De Conno, F., Caraceni, A., Aldrighetti, L. *et al.* (1993) Paraplegia following coeliac plexus block. *Pain*, **55**, 383–385.

De Leon-Casasola, O.A., Kent, E. and Lema, M.J. (1993) Neurolytic superior hypogastric plexus block for chronic pelvic pain associated with cancer. *Pain*, **54**, 145–151.

Ellershaw, J.E., Wilkinson, P., Duncan, T. *et al.* (1996) Is there a role for neural blockade in the control of unrelieved pain in hospice in patients? *Palliat. Med.* **10**, 61.

Kalso, E., Heiskanen, T., Rantio, M. *et al.* (1996) Epidural and subcutaneous morphine in the management of cancer pain: a double-blind crossover study. *Pain*, **67**(2–3), 443–449.

Krames, E.S. (1993) The chronic intraspinal use of opioid and local anaesthetic mixtures for the relief of intractable pain: when all else fails! *Pain*, **55**, 1–4.

Makin, W. and Regnard, C. (1994) An audit of spinal analgesia for the pain of advanced cancer. *Palliat. Med.*, **8**(1), 75.

Mercadante, S. (1993) Coeliac plexus block versus analgesics in pancreatic cancer pain. *Pain*, *52*(2), 187–192.

Stuart, G. and Cramond, T. (1993) Role of percutaneous cervical cordotomy for pain of malignant origin. *Med. J. Australia*, **158**, 667–670.

Van Dongen, R.T.M., Crul, B.J.P. and De Bock, M. (1993) Long-term intrathecal infusion of morphine and morphine/bupivacaine mixtures in the treatment of cancer pain: a retrospective analysis of 51 cases. *Pain*, **55**, 119–123.

Van Dongen, R.T.M., Van, EeR and Crul, B.J. (1997) Neurological impairment during long-term intrathecal infusion of bupivacaine in cancer patients: a sign of spinal cord compression. *Pain*, **69**, 205–209.

Neuropathic pain

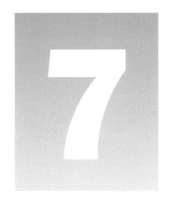

There are few problems in palliative medicine that can be so difficult to diagnose and treat as neuropathic pain, and none more satisfying if the outcome is a patient who is pain free and remains so. The difficulties, however, are often multiple. When a nerve is damaged by an insult such as trauma to the brachial plexus or herpes zoster upon a peripheral nerve, the damage sustained is precise, accurately localized, affects no other tissues, is clearly identified by some incident in the past, remains static or possibly slowly improves with time and is therefore a 'pure' neuropathy. In cancer, on the other hand, the pathology is not confined to nerves but affects many other tissues simultaneously. The pain can therefore be part neuropathic, part nociceptive. Some of it may respond to an opioid, some to an NSAID, some perhaps to immobilizing a limb or to treatment with high-dose steroids. However, a neuropathic component that requires different treatment can still remain. Furthermore, the pathology is not static but remorselessly progressive, so that treatments that were effective a month ago are now totally or partially without benefit. Also the general condition of the patient is often deteriorating, so other organs begin to fail, emaciation becomes a problem and the patient's deteriorating health can heighten his or her awareness of pain and increase demands for rapid relief.

Neuropathic pain can be defined as pain arising from disturbance of function or pathological change in the peripheral or central nervous system, and can be caused by compression or infiltration of nerves by a tumour. It can be recognized if the pain is distributed in a way that is consistent with neural damage and if there is evidence of corresponding neural injury (Martin and Hagen, 1997). These abnormalities can be described as allodynia, a sensation of pain evoked by stimulus that does not normally provoke pain in an area of altered sensation, or as hyperalgesia, which is a disproportionately severe pain sensation in response to a noxious stimulus. There may also be hyperpathia, which is an exaggerated reaction often of an explosive nature after a normally pain-producing stimulus or a stimulus that normally produces another sensation. The abnormal sensation experienced may be tingling, prickling, electric shocks, burning or shooting lancinating pain.

In addition to the abnormal sensations being experienced in peripheral nerve territories the central nervous system displays a great ability to react to the stimuli that are being received by intensifying and prolonging them. This phenomenon known as 'wind up' (Ren Ke, 1994), can be produced under laboratory conditions in which repeated stimulation causes an increased response in the spinal cord greater in amplitude than would otherwise be expected, and which lasts for a considerable time after the initiating stimulus has ceased.

In making a diagnosis of neuropathic pain it is essential to record exactly what the patient is experiencing, both the type and the severity of the pain, using the patient's exact words without prompting wherever possible. The presence of severe pain resulting from light touch from a hand, clothing or sheets is highly significant. Because pain and temperature are very closely related sensations it is worth checking whether the patient can detect the difference between warm and cold objects applied to the skin. Boiling water and ice are not necessary. A normal object that is readily available in the home is perfectly satisfactory to detect the change, and if temperature sensation is abnormal this is a highly significant finding. It should be possible to demonstrate clinically that the abnormal sensation is being experienced in the territory of a peripheral nerve or of a dermatome, which may be single or multiple if a large area is affected. Physical examination should also include simple tests for eliciting pain in peripheral nerves. The straight leg raising test for sciatic nerve involvement is of limited value; far better is the slump test, when the patient sits with neck bowed forward and hands behind the back. The knee is then gently extended to stretch the sciatic nerve fully and if at some point in its course it is involved by tumour the patient will actively resist further extension. Similarly, to stretch the femoral nerve the patient should lie face down and the knee is then steadily flexed to bring the heel towards the buttock. If the femoral nerve is invaded at any point in its course, the patient will actively resist this manoeuvre and describe the typical pain running down the front of the thigh to the patella.

Investigations are often required to determine the level of the patho-logical changes. X-rays are of limited help unless there is erosion or collapse of spinal vertebrae. CT scans are often helpful and MRI studies invaluable in visualizing the nature and extent of the disease.

Treatment

Traditionally it was claimed that neuropathic pain was resistant to opioids. However, this is not a clear-cut distinction that is helpful in clinical practice. Because much of the pain experienced in a metastatic cancer is not

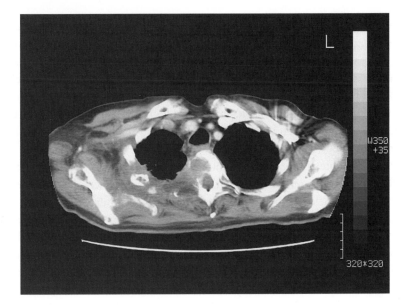

Figure 7.1
CT scan showing a carcinoma of lung in a patient with Pancoast's syndrome. There is extensive erosion of the right fourth and third ribs posteriorly, with erosion of the pedicle of the third thoracic vertebra and extension of the tumour into the spinal cord.

neuropathic there may well be considerable improvement resulting from the use of opioids. For example, Figure 7.1 shows a carcinoma of lung in a patient with extensive infiltration of the brachial plexus, third and fourth ribs, third thoracic vertebra and spinal canal due to a Pancoast tumour, who was completely pain free on MST 30 mg bd plus an NSAID. Opioids are believed to reduce, if not abolish, some neuropathic pains when tested in post-herpetic neuralgia and in other non-malignant situations. It is therefore always worth while trying a strong opioid first until side-effects make further increases impossible. One then moves to the adjuvant analgesics. These can be grouped into the tricyclic antidepressants such as amitriptyline, desipramine and nortriptyline, the anticonvulsants, particularly carbamazepine and sodium valproate and oral local anaesthetics such as mexiletine and flecainide. The anaesthetic agent ketamine is also an effective analgesic in sub-anaesthetic doses.

THE TRICYCLIC ANTIDEPRESSANTS

The role of antidepressants has been systematically reviewed by McQuay *et al.* (1996). In a review of 17 randomized controlled trials (but not involving cancer patients) they found that 30% of patients so treated obtained more than 50% pain relief, 30% had minor adverse reactions and 4% had to stop treatment because of major adverse effects. There was no agreement on the best antidepressant to use but there was a clear bias in favour of the older tricyclic group rather than newer drugs such as paroxetine and mianserin.

In clinical practice amitriptyline is used as the first tricyclic antidepressant to be tried, starting with a dose of 10 mg at night. Sometimes this is sufficient and when it works the benefit is almost immediate. The outcome is not in any way related to the mental state of the patient, for tricyclics work not by relieving depression but by enhancing the inhibitory impulses at spinal cord level which block pain physiologically. It is believed that this effect is due to their action in enhancing the adrenergic synaptic connections.

If amitriptyline 10 mg at night is not sufficient, the dose is steadily increased until either the pain remits or the patient develops side-effects. These are more common in the elderly and typically are increasing confusion, sedation, dry mouth and blurred vision. Amitriptyline can be cumulative; therefore the same daily dose may give increasing benefits and side-effects over a week or 10 days. Bowsher (1994) found that if he reached the limit of tolerability in patients with post-herpetic neuralgia the effect of amitriptyline could be enhanced by adding dexamphetamine 10 mg tds. He believed that this increased the adrenergic effects in the spinal cord synapses.

Desipramine is less sedative than amitriptyline and may be preferable if it causes less side-effects. In a study comparing desipramine with amitriptyline and fluoxetine it was found to have similar efficacy to amitriptyline but quite markedly less side-effects. Fluoxetine was no more effective than a placebo (Max *et al.*, 1992). It is therefore possible to push the dose of desipramine to a higher level and in theory to obtain better results if the side-effects are less. Unfortunately, this drug is available in Great Britain only to order on a named patient basis. In a study by Eija, Tinna and Pertti (1995) amitriptyline was given to patients with metastatic breast cancer in a randomized double-blind placebo-controlled cross-over study of 15 patients. The dose was escalated from 25 mg to 100 mg daily over 4 weeks. The active treatment significantly relieved neuropathic pain both in the arm and around the breast scar. Eight out of 15 patients had more than a 50% decrease in pain intensity. However, the authors comment that the adverse effects of amitriptyline put most of the patients off from using the drug regularly. Tiredness and dry mouth were particularly distressing for patients on 50 mg a day and for patients taking 100 mg daily constipation and sweating were also significantly more common than for those patients on placebo. Only 20% of the patients treated wanted to continue taking amitriptyline after the trial was completed. Similar findings were reported by McQuay, Carroll and Glynn (1993) where patients on 25, 50 and 75 mg per day were compared. The highest dose provides significantly greater efficacy but also a significantly higher incidence of side-effects.

In theory nortriptyline should be as effective as amitriptyline because it is the active drug in vivo to which amitriptyline is metabolized. It is much less sedative than amitriptyline. However, it has been little studied and no convincing double-blind trials have been reported to show its effectiveness or superiority. A recent review (McQuay and Moore, 1997) could give no evidence that one drug was better than another, though the authors advocated changing drugs to avoid adverse effects. Another review article could find no evidence that tricyclics other than amitriptyline were effective (Sykes, Johnson and Hanks, 1997).

THE ANTICONVULSANTS

If treatment with tricyclic antidepressants fails or is blocked by side-effects, then most clinicians will move to the use of an anticonvulsant. It is postulated that much neuropathic pain, particularly the shooting lancinating type, is caused by abnormal electrical discharges from damaged nerve fibres. A drug that inhibits electrical discharge does therefore have theoretical reasons for its use. For treating trigeminal neuralgia carbamazepine is the drug of choice, and is commonly effective with other neuropathies. Unfortunately, it causes marked sedation and confusion, particularly in the elderly, and is only tolerated by many if the dose is escalated very gradually. Our routine is to start with 100 mg bd and gradually increase the dosage at 4–7 day intervals until either the pain remits or side-effects become intolerable. In a systematic review of anticonvulsants in neuropathic pain McQuay *et al.* (1995) found only one trial that was concerned with cancer pain. This compared buprenorphine alone with phenytoin and both drugs together. The combination treatment was considered to be the best. No placebo-controlled trial was found that could prove the analgesic effects of sodium valproate, yet this drug is commonly used for analgesia if carbamazepine proves ineffective or intolerable. A dose of 200 mg tds is usual, with titration upwards until the patient is pain free or side-effects supervene.

OTHER DRUG TREATMENTS

If tricyclic antidepressants and anticonvulsants fail to relieve neuropathic pain, there is no clear option for a third-line drug. In hospices with an efficient and effective anaesthetic service many clinicians will proceed rapidly to either an epidural or more commonly now an intrathecal spinal line (p. 56). Mexiletine has been claimed to relieve neuropathic pain in rats (Jett *et al.*, 1997), but it can have serious cardiovascular side-effects, which make many clinicians wary of employing it. Galer, Harle and Rowbotham (1996) used the local anaesthetic lidocaine in nine patients to predict whether or not they would respond to subsequent treatment with oral mexiletine. Both 2 mg/kg and 5 mg/kg lidocaine infused intravenously over

45 minutes significantly reduced neuropathic pain as measured by the VAS score. Subsequent response to oral mexiletine was significantly correlated with the average response to the two doses of lidocaine.

Clonidine

In a series of 85 patients with severe cancer pain who were either unrelieved by large doses of opioids or developed side-effects that limited the dosage, treatment was changed to epidural clonidine 30 µg/hour or placebo for 14 days together with rescue doses of epidural morphine. The primary pain was judged to be neuropathic in 36 patients and non-neuropathic in the other 49 patients, but 70 patients had a second and 37 patients a third pain as well. Almost half of both groups failed to complete the full 14 day treatment course. Clonidine produced a higher success rate than placebo (45% versus 21%) due almost entirely to a large difference in success rate in patients with neuropathic pain. The commonest side-effect encountered was hypotension either at rest (45%) or standing (32%). Other side-effects did not vary from or were less than those encountered by patients on a placebo. Only two patients were seriously affected by decreased blood pressure (Eisenach et al., 1995).

Ketamine

As mentioned earlier, ketamine is an old anaesthetic agent whose use has been largely discontinued, except in children, because of the intense dysphoria it produces in many patients after recovery from its anaesthetic effects. However, at low doses it has potent analgesic activity. It is believed to inhibit the NMDA receptor mechanism, so blocking neuropathic pain and preventing 'wind up'. It has been suggested that there is a synergistic effect between ketamine and opioids (Mercadante, 1996). Certainly ketamine can rescue clinicians from situations of overwhelming pain where all other therapeutic options have been tried or are not possible (Laird and Lovel, 1993). Ketamine has also been used in non-malignant neuropathic pain, particularly in the mouth and face (Mathisen et al., 1995). They compared the analgesic effect of racemic ketamine and its two enantiomers in 16 female patients in acute pain after oral surgery and in seven female patients with chronic neuropathic orofacial pain. They found all three forms of ketamine consistently relieved post-operative pain, S(+) ketamine being four times more potent than R(−) ketamine. The mental side-effects, i.e. dysphoria, were qualitatively similar with the three forms but with regard to the analgesic effect S(+) ketamine caused more disturbing side-effects than did R(−) ketamine. They support the view that ketamine inhibits the NMDA receptors and that therefore these receptors are important in the perception of acute pain.

Luczak *et al.* (1995) similarly reported marked success in 32 patients with cancer when other methods failed. They gave it orally in doses ranging from 10 to 50 mg every 4 hours or subcutaneously in doses of 50–700 mg per 24 hours together with morphine, and to prevent psychomimetic side-effects 19 patients also received either diazepam or midazolam. Very good or good pain relief was achieved in 24 patients (75%) and partial benefit in a further six patients. In six patients the addition of ketamine to previous treatment led to a reduction of the dose of morphine by 40–80%. Two patients reported bad dreams which were prevented by haloperidol 3 mg nocte. Four patients reported drowsiness. Respiratory depression was not seen. The authors felt that a benzodiazepine would prevent dysphoria. They recommended starting ketamine in a palliative care ward under experienced professional supervision, starting with small doses of 5 mg intravenously, monitoring vital signs and having naloxone prepared in a syringe before the first dose in case the morphine sparing effect produced marked respiratory depression after the ketamine injection. They proposed that ketamine could be considered as the fourth step of the WHO analgesic ladder.

A double-blind multi-dose trial of ketamine 0–40 mg intramuscularly eight times per day added to intramuscular morphine therapy was given to a 61-year-old man with a chronic back pain due to osteoporosis (Cherry *et al.*, 1995). The patient reported only mild side-effects and pain scores 30 minutes after doses were significantly reduced in a dose-related manner. The amount of morphine used by the patient was significantly reduced as the ketamine dose was increased. Although only a single patient is described here, this *N* of 1 trial demonstrated benefit to the patient without the need to give a placebo to a patient in severe distress.

References

Bowsher, D. (1994) Post-herpetic neuralgia in older patients: incidence and optimal treatment. *Drugs & Aging*, 5(6), 411–418.

Cherry, D.A., Plummer, J.L., Gourley, G.K. *et al.* (1995). Ketamine as an adjunct to morphine in the treatment of pain. *Pain*, **62**, 119–121.

Eija, K., Tiina, T. and Pertti, N. (1995) Amitriptyline effectively relieves neuropathic pain following treatment of breast cancer. *Pain*, **64**, 293–302.

Eisenach, J.C., Dupen, S., Dubois, M. *et al.* (1995) Epidural clonidine analgesia for intractable cancer pain. *Pain*, **61**, 391–399.

Galer, B.S., Harle, J. and Rowbotham, M.C. (1996) Response to intravenous lidocaine infusion predicts subsequent response to oral mexiletine: a prospective study. *J. Pain Symp. Manage.*, **12**(3), 161–167.

Jett, M.F., McGuirk, J., Waligora, D. and Hunter, J.C. (1997) The effects of mexiletine, desipramine and fluoxetine in rat models involving central sensitization. *Pain*, **69**(1–2), 161–169.

Laird, D. and Lovel, T.W.I. (1993) Paradoxical pain. *Lancet*, **341**(8839), 241.

Luczak, J., Dickenson, A.H. and Kotlinska-Lemieszek, A. (1995) The role of ketamine, an NMDA receptor antagonist, in the management of pain. *Prog. Palliative Care*, **3**(4), 127–134.

Martin, L.A. and Hagen, N.A. (1997) Neuropathic pain in cancer patients: mechanisms, syndromes, and clinical controversies. *J. Pain Symp. Manage.*, **14**(2), 99–117.

Mathisen, L.C., Skjelbred, P., Skoglund, L.A. and Øye I. (1995) Effect of ketamine, an NMDA receptor inhibitor, in acute and chronic orofacial pain. *Pain*, **61**, 215–220.

Max, M.B., Lynch, S.A., Muir, J. *et al.* (1992) *N. Engl. J. Med.*, **326**(19), 1250–1255.

Mercadante S. (1996) Ketamine in cancer pain: an update. *Palliat. Med.*, **10**, 225–230.

McQuay, H.J. and Moore, R.A. (1997) Antidepressants and chronic pain. *Br. Med. J.*, **314**, 763–764.

McQuay, H.J., Carroll, D. and Glynn, C.J. (1993) Dose-response for analgesic effect of amitriptyline in chronic pain. *Anaesthesia*, **48**, 281–285.

McQuay, H.J., Carroll, D., Jadad, A.R. *et al.* (1995) Anticonvulsant drugs for management of pain: a systematic review. *Br. Med. J.*, **311**, 1047–1051.

McQuay, H.J., Tramer, M., Nye, B.A. *et al.* (1996) A systematic review of antidepressants in neuropathic pain. *Pain*, **68**, 217–227.

Ren Ke. (1994) Wind-up and the NMDA receptor: from animal studies to humans. *Pain*, **59**, 157–158.

Sykes, J., Johnson, R. and Hanks, G.W. (1997) Difficult pain problems. *Br. Med. J.*, **315**, 867–869.

Corticosteroids for the relief of pain

It is well known that the corticosteroid group of drugs can reduce the size of some tumours and that the pain caused by them is thereby reduced or abolished. In space-occupying tumours within the skull the use of steroids is routine in abolishing the headache, photophobia and impaired cognitive function. This benefit can result whether the tumour is a primary glioma or a metastasis from a primary carcinoma elsewhere. The change can be dramatic, often within hours or even minutes of giving the corticosteroid, particularly if it is administered intravenously. The patient can almost wake up on the point of the needle from a near moribund state to full consciousness. The steroid usually employed is dexamethasone because it is by far the most powerful and predictable in its effect. Depending on body size, the usual dose given is 16–24 mg per 24 hours. It is best given in a single morning dose, for otherwise it greatly disturbs the normal sleep pattern. Dexamethasone has a very long half-life in the body, so its beneficial effects will last for much longer than 24 hours.

Less well known is the effect of dexamethasone upon pain in the liver. Liver tissue itself suffers no pain but the enclosing capsule is made of peritoneum and is exquisitely sensitive to irritation and to stretching. Therefore if the liver is grossly enlarged by widespread hepatic metastases, the capsule is stretched to perhaps three or four times its normal size. Also, if the tumour is eroding through the surface, it will directly irritate and eventually break through the peritoneal capsule. This can give rise to severe pain classically referred to the right shoulder tip. Such liver capsule pain is notoriously resistant to treatment with opioids, but it will respond, again often in dramatic fashion, to dexamethasone. The same dose is used as with intracranial tumours. It is traditional to give prophylactic treatment to prevent gastric erosion and haemorrhage. Patients having transplants who are treated with steroids for long periods are given cimetidine 200 mg tds and it is claimed that gastrointestinal complications are negligible. However, this has not been subjected to a formal trial in cancer patients. In neurosurgery, steroids plus cimetidine and an antacid have reduced gastro-intestinal bleeding from eight patients out of 15 on antacid only to three patients out of 17 (P = 0.03) (Tibbs *et al.*, 1981). Misoprostol as prophylaxis is well proven for use with NSAIDs but its benefits when given with steroids are unknown. The benefit from omeprazole is also unknown (Ellershaw and Kelly, 1994). The same authors derived a risk factor based upon the total dose of steroids given (i e. the amount and the length of treatment), a past history of peptic ulcer, the presence of advanced malignant disease and the concurrent administration of an NSAID. They concluded that two or more of these risk factors indicate the need to give prophylaxis. They also proposed that there is a severe danger of complications if the total dose of steroid given is greater than 1000 mg of prednisolone or 140 mg of dexamethasone.

Whatever prophylaxis is given it is prudent to reduce the dose as quickly as possible to the minimum effective level. One needs to know quickly whether corticosteroids are going to help the patient's symptoms and therefore it is legitimate to start with a high dose. If after four or five days there has been no benefit, the steroids can be acutely stopped because the patient will not be steroid dependent after so short a time. If the high dose works then the dosage should be progressively reduced by 2 mg per day or 4 mg on alternate days to the least possible effective level. This can be quite specific; a patient with headache due to intracerebral malignancy may be completely comfortable on 6 mg of dexamethasone a day and incapacitated by headache on 4 mg per day. Titration of the dose to the symptoms is therefore mandatory.

It is not known how corticosteroids work in these situations. With brain tumours it was traditional to claim that peritumour oedema had been reduced, thus giving more space for the tumour to expand. There is no good evidence for this. It is claimed that in both the brain and the liver dexamethasone works by expelling volumes of blood from the large venous sinuses in both organs, so making more space and reducing the pressure within the skull or within the liver capsule. This is equally unproven. Whatever the mechanism, corticosteroids are invaluable in these situations.

Dexamethasone is also used acutely to try to avert paraplegia when patients have a spread of malignant tissue within the spinal canal. If this can be shrunk, the cord may be saved for long enough for emergency radiotherapy to the affected area to have a chance to work. The dose of dexamethasone usually employed is 24–32 mg and some radiotherapists advocate a dose as high as 96 mg to avert disaster. There is no evidence that such heroic doses confer any greater benefit than the standard level.

Corticosteroids are also often used, and are sometimes effective, in reducing pressure in other situations. Compression or distortion of the brachial plexus or lumbosacral plexus due to malignancy can cause severe neuropathic pain in the arm or leg, respectively, and sometimes high-dose steroids will give a worthwhile, though temporary, result. Tumours in the neck, e.g. metastases from carcinoma of larynx, can also sometimes shrink dramatically, as can some lymphomas.

Case report

A 71-year-old woman with metastatic carcinoma of larynx was referred for terminal care. Chemotherapy had been ineffective and radiotherapy had shrunk the tumour masses for some months, though they had since regrown. She was greatly distressed by their presence, for the whole neck was encircled by a massive ring of tumour extending from the clavicles almost up to the angle of the jaw. Her face was plethoric, with protruding eyeballs and injected conjunctivae, because there was almost complete obstruction of the venous return from the head. High-dose dexamethasone (32 mg per day) produced a dramatic shrinking of the tumour, the engorgement resolved and the patient was enormously grateful. The steroid dose was progressively reduced to 6 mg a day and she lived for another 2 weeks in comfort. The tumour then began to regrow and a second treatment with high-dose steroids failed to produce the same benefit. An attempt to stent the jugular veins was unsuccessful and the patient died from a myocardial infarct shortly afterwards.

Other indications for using corticosteroids to relieve pain include metastatic arthralgia and obstruction of bronchus, ureter and possibly intestine.

Apart from peptic ulceration and bleeding, the other side-effects of corticosteroids are well known. They include diabetes, osteoporosis, paranoid psychosis, muscle wasting, particularly of the proximal muscles around the pelvis, and the development of a typical Cushing's syndrome. The myopathy is probably the most frequently encountered side-effect of prolonged steroid treatment in cancer patients. Typically the patient notices that walking upstairs is becoming difficult and has increasing difficulty in getting out of a chair, even though once erect he or she can walk perfectly well. This occurs long before wasting of peripheral muscles can be detected, and is a symptom that requires urgent reduction of steroids if possible if the patient is not to become severely disabled. The most dramatic side-effect is undoubtedly the development of an acute psychotic reaction which can be terrifying in its severity and rapid onset. The only effective treatment is to stop the steroids immediately and give chlorpromazine over several days until the effects of the corticosteroid are eliminated. Maintenance treatment with hydrocortisone may be required to prevent acute adrenal insufficiency.

The use of corticosteroids for pain relief (and other benefits) is reviewed by Twycross (1994).

References

Ellershaw, J.E. and Kelly, M.J. (1994) Corticosteroids and peptic ulceration. *Palliat. Med.*, **8**(4), 313–319.

Twycross, R. (1994) *Pain Relief in Advanced Cancer*, Churchill Livingstone, Edinburgh.

Other pains and treatments

Cramp

Almost everybody experiences cramp at some time or another. Some people who are otherwise healthy experience cramp usually in the calf muscles or the feet very frequently, others get it occasionally, particularly after exertion and sometimes following alcoholic excess. The standard treatment is quinine bisulphate at night 300 mg. The reason for its effect is unknown but it is very commonly effective. Quinine is normally well tolerated but can rarely produce thrombocytopenia and in excess can produce a syndrome of vomiting, tinnitus and deafness (Connolly *et al.*, 1992). However, patients with cancer can develop pain in muscles and in fascia which they may often call cramp and which is often associated with proximity of the affected muscles to bony metastases. Another cause can be involvement of nerve roots or side-effects from drugs, particularly some hormones.

Sometimes cramp is associated with the presence of trigger points which can be palpated in the muscle and will when pressed produce pain, often associated with a jump that the patient feels. With trigger points the pain is brought on by the use of the muscle in question and the diagnostic feature is that injection of local anaesthetic into the trigger point eliminates both the pain and tenderness. The treatment consists of repeating the local anaesthetic injection until the pain is permanently relieved. Physiotherapy is also often helpful.

Headache

Patients with disseminated cancer very frequently complain of headache and its onset is always a symptom to be treated seriously. Clearly both patient and clinician will be worried that the onset of headache indicates the presence of intracerebral metastases causing raised intracranial pressure, and this is quite frequently so. The patient may also have associated symptoms of photophobia, neck stiffness together with retardation of thought processes, and sometimes focal neurological signs together with obvious papilloedema. Treatment of headache from this cause is dealt with on p. 67.

However, not infrequently patients complain bitterly of headache when papilloedema and other signs of raised intracranial pressure are not present. This can lead the clinician into the unwise belief that because there is no rise in intracranial pressure there can be no malignant disease. This is far from the case. Sometimes tumours within the brain cause pain without raising the pressure, while in other cases, particularly in the posterior fossa, the tumour may not be visualized on CT scanning until it is quite large.

Table 9.1

Pain syndromes caused by invasion of skull

Syndrome	Pathophysiology	Characteristics of pain	Concomitants
Cavernous sinus	Metastasis to cavernous sinus	Frontal headache	Dysfunction of cranial nerves III–VI (diplopia, ophthalmoplegia, papilloedema)
Sphenoid sinus	Metastasis to the sphenoid sinus	Frontal headache radiating to temple with intermittent retro-orbital pain	Dysfunction of cranial nerve VI (diplopia) and nasal stuffiness
Clivus syndrome	Metastasis to clivus of sphenoid bone and basilar part of occipital bone	Vertex headache exacerbated by neck flexion	Dysfunction of cranial nerves VII and IX–XII (facial weakness, hoarseness, dysarthria, dysphagia, trapezius muscle weakness). Begins unilaterally but extends bilaterally
Jugular foramen	Metastasis to jugular foramen	Occipital pain exacerbated by head movement, radiating to the vertex and to shoulder and arm	Dysfunction of cranial nerves IX–XII (hoarseness, dysarthria, dysphagia, trapezius muscle weakness)
Occipital condyle	Metastasis to occipital condyle	Localized occipital pain exacerbated by neck flexion	Dysfunction of cranial nerve XII (paralysis of tongue → dysarthria and buccal dysphagia), weakness of sternomastoid muscle, stiff neck

Sources: Foley, 1979; Portenoy, 1989; Bonica, 1990. Reprinted with permission from R.G. Twycross, *Pain Relief in Advanced Cancer*, Churchill Livingstone, 1994.

Furthermore, malignant infiltration of the meninges and the sinuses of the skull may give rise to specific headache syndromes without raising the pressure within the skull. Such syndromes are characteristic and are summarized in Table 9.1.

Treatment of headache is frequently difficult. Raised intracranial pressure will respond to high dose dexamethasone (p. 68), and sometimes if hydrocephalus is present due to blockage of the aqueduct or fourth ventricle, it may be necessary to put in a shunt from one lateral ventricle to the venous system. This can be dramatically successful in relieving otherwise intolerable headache. Debulking of large tumours is helpful, as is palliative radiotherapy.

When headache is due to infiltration of the bones of the skull palliative radiotherapy and analgesics are the mainstay of treatment. An NSAID such as diclofenac should always be tried first and only if this is not completely successful should moderate or strong opioids be used. Radiotherapy should be offered and in theory intravenous treatment with bisphosphonates such as pamidronate might well be helpful if bone involvement is extensive.

Transcutaneous electrical nerve stimulation (TENS)

The application of electric stimuli to relieve pain has a very long and respectable history going back to the time of Hypocrates, who used electric fish. In modern times the 'gate' theory that pain can be blocked by the activity of nervous impulses in the spinal cord reawakened the idea that such blocking could be induced by external means. Machines were therefore produced with the aim of stimulating the dorsal columns of the spinal cord or the peripheral nerves proximal to the site of the pain (Figure 9.1). Electrodes, which are either disposable or reusable, are applied to the skin. Originally jelly was required to obtain a good electrical conduction, but nowadays Polymor pads are preferable and need no jelly or tapes to hold them on. They are applied to the dermatome affected by pain proximal to the lesion (Figure 9.2) and treatment is given either continuously or as impulses. The patient needs to be reassured that repeated use is harmless and indeed can be switched on and off at will. At least a month's trial should be undertaken before it can be decided whether or not the treatment is effective. Trial and error is essential, and the assistance of an experienced physiotherapist gives a much better chance of success. The machines are widely available and not expensive. It is important that the electrodes are applied to the correct dermatome and that they are proximal to the site of the pain. The stimulus should be strong but comfortable and not taken to

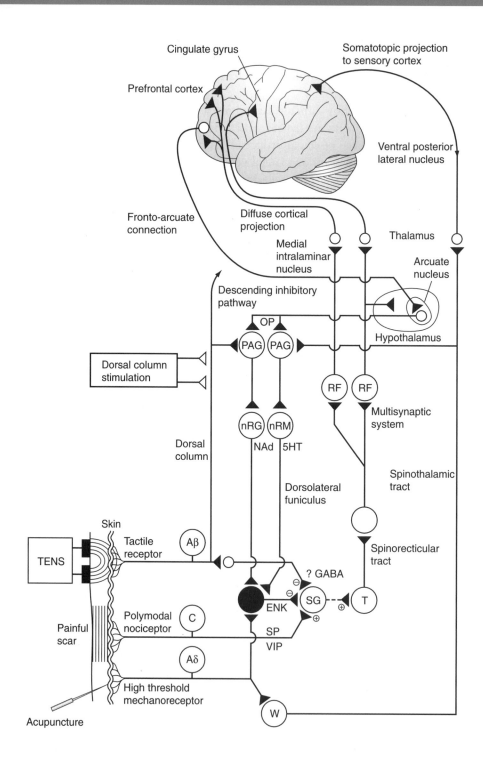

the limits of toleration. Muscle twitching or spasm should not be produced (unless the acupuncture-like mode is deliberately being employed).

Clinical trials have been reported that show that the benefits of TENS are more than would be expected from a placebo and it is a form of treatment which is well worth trying, in addition to conventional analgesic drugs. Some patients are completely unresponsive, while in others after an initial benefit tolerance appears to occur, which ends the usefulness of the treatment (Table 9.2).

TENS should not be used on pregnant women.

Acupuncture

This method of treatment for relief of pain has an even longer history than electrical stimulation. Its origins are lost in the history of Chinese medicine, but both traditional Chinese acupuncture and Western acupuncture have become well accepted for producing analgesia in selected patients. Few controlled clinical trials exist to confirm the effectiveness of acupuncture and although uncontrolled trials of this treatment give a 50–70% successful response rate, this is poor-quality evidence. In placebo-controlled surveys, however, most results favour acupuncture over placebo, though the success rate does not attain that of uncontrolled studies. It is difficult to devise an adequate placebo and therefore really well designed trials of high quality are extremely difficult to set up. A skilled practitioner of either Chinese or Western models of treatment can help some patients enormously and a larger number to a lesser extent. Again, the control of pain by acupuncture is well worth a trial in patients receiving standard conventional medical treatment. For more detailed discussion of methods and of the neuropharmacological justification for TENS and acupuncture see Thompson and Filshie (1998).

Figure 9.1

Diagram to show neuronal circuits involved in TENS and acupuncture analgesia. The afferent pathways involved in transmitting nociceptive information from a painful scar to the higher centres via the dorsal horn, the ascending tracts, and the thalamus are shown. The connections to the descending inhibitory pathways which descend in the dorsolateral funiculus are also shown. The connections to the hypothalamus are indicated. Abbreviations $A\beta$, C, and $A\delta$ represent the posterior root ganglion cells of $A\beta$, C, and $A\delta$ fibres, respectively; SP = substance P; VIP = vasoactive intestinal polypeptide; GABA = γ-aminobutyric acid; OP = opioid peptides; SG = cell in the substantia gelatinosa (lamina II); ENK = enkephalinergic neurone; T = transmission cell; W = Waldeyer cell; PAG = periaqueductal grey; nRG = cell in the nucleus raphe gigantocellularis; hRM = cell in the nucleus raphe magnus; NAd = noradrenaline; 5-HT = 5-hydroxytryptamine. Reprinted with permission from D. Doyle, W.C. Hanks & N. MacDonald, *Oxford Textbook of Palliative Medicine*, Second Edition, Oxford University Press, 1998.

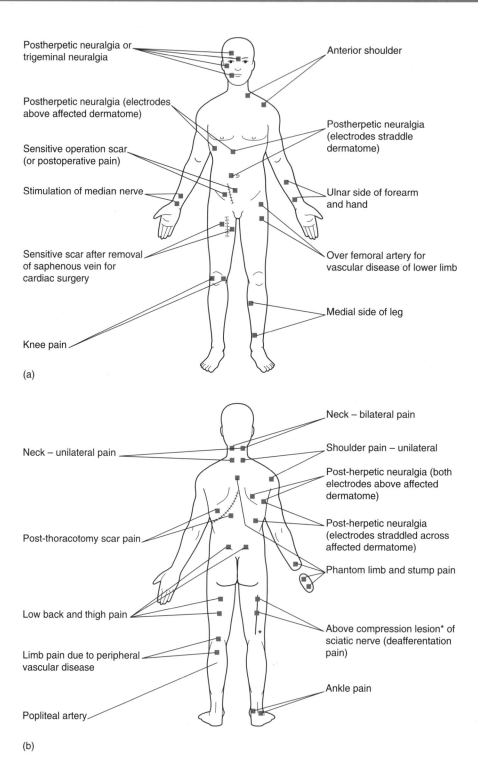

Postherpetic neuralgia or trigeminal neuralgia

Anterior shoulder

Postherpetic neuralgia (electrodes above affected dermatome)

Postherpetic neuralgia (electrodes straddle dermatome)

Sensitive operation scar (or postoperative pain)

Stimulation of median nerve

Ulnar side of forearm and hand

Sensitive scar after removal of saphenous vein for cardiac surgery

Over femoral artery for vascular disease of lower limb

Medial side of leg

Knee pain

(a)

Neck – bilateral pain

Neck – unilateral pain

Shoulder pain – unilateral

Post-herpetic neuralgia (both electrodes above affected dermatome)

Post-herpetic neuralgia (electrodes straddled across affected dermatome)

Post-thoracotomy scar pain

Phantom limb and stump pain

Low back and thigh pain

Above compression lesion* of sciatic nerve (deafferentation pain)

Limb pain due to peripheral vascular disease

Ankle pain

Popliteal artery

(b)

Author	Good or complete pain relief	Partial pain relief or reduction of analgesics	No relief	Total (comments)
Long (1974)	3 (60%)	–	2 (40%)	5 malignancies out of total series of 197 cases
Hardy (1975)	2 (50%)	–	2 (50%)	4 out of 53
Loeser et al. (1975)	–	3 (42%)	4 (57%)	7 out of 198
Campbell and Long (1976)	1 (25%)	–	3 (75%)	4
Ostrowski (1979)	4 (44%)	4 (44%)	1 (11%)	9
Ventafridda (1979)	36 (97%) 1–10 days 4 (11%) at 30 days	–	1 (3%) 33 (89%) at 30 days	37 37
Bates and Nathan (1980)	4 (80%) (all longer than 1 week)	–	1 (20%)	5
Avellanosa and West (1982)				
2 weeks	17 (28%)	22 (37%)	21 (35%)	60
3 months	9 (15%)	11 (18%)	40 (67%)	60
Dil-din et al. (1985)	11 (100%)	–	–	11 (abstract only available)
Rafter (1986) [quoted by Librach and Rapson (1988)] Range	15–99%	2–44%	3–75%	

Reprinted with permission from D. Doyle, W.C. Hanks & N. MacDonald, *Oxford Textbook of Palliative Medicine*, Second Edition, Oxford Universty Press, 1998.

There is no doubt that some patients are greatly helped by either TENS or acupuncture and sometimes by both. Both are well worth trying in obtaining relief for the objective and subjective sensations that our patients suffer and deserve a trial in any situation where pain control is less than perfect.

Table 9.2

TENS for the treatment of malignant disease

Figure 9.2

Drawing of electrode positions commonly used for TENS. (a) Anterior aspect. (b) Posterior aspect. (Reprinted with permission from D. Doyle, W.C. Hanks & N. MacDonald, *Oxford Textbook of Palliative Medicine*, 2nd edn, Oxford University Press, 1998.

References

Avellanosa, A.M. and West, C.R. (1982) Experience with transcutaneous nerve stimulation for relief of intractable pain in cancer patients. *J. Med*, **13**, 203–213.

Bates, J.A.V. and Nathan, P.W. (1980) Transcutaneous electrical nerve stimulation for chronic pain. *Anaesthesia*, **35**, 817–822.

Bonica, J.J. (1990) *The Management of Pain*, 2nd edn, Lea & Febiger, Philadelphia.

Campbell, J.N. and Long, D.M. (1976) Peripheral nerve stimulation in the treatment of intractable pain. *J. Neurosurg*, **45**, 692–699.

Connolly, P.S., Shirley, E.A., Wasson, J.H. and Nierenberg, D.W. (1992) The treatment of nocturnal leg cramps: a cross-over trial of quinine v. vitamin E. *Arch. Int. Med.*

Dil-din, A.S., Tikhonova, G.P. and Kozov, S.V. (1985) Transcutaneous electro-stimulation method leading to a permeation system of electro-analgesia in oncological practice. *Vopr-Onkologica*, **31**, 33–36.

Foley, K.M. (1979) Pain syndromes in patients with cancer, in *Advances in Pain Research and Therapy*, vol. 2 (eds J.J. Bonica and V. Ventafridda), pp. 59–75, Raven Press, New York.

Hardy, R.W. (1975) Current techniques in the management of pain. *Cleveland Clinical Quarterly*, **41**, 177–183.

Librach, S.I. and Rapson, L.M. (1988) The use of transcutaneous electrical nerve stimulation (TENS) for the relief of pain in palliative care. *Palliat. Med.*, **2**, 15–20.

Loeser, J.D., Black, R.G. and Christman, A. (1975) Relief of pain by transcutaneous stimulation. *J. Neurosurg.*, **42**, 308–314.

Long, D.M. (1974) External electrical stimulation as a treatment of chronic pain. *Minnesota Medicine*, **57**, 195–198.

Ostrowski, M.J. (1979) Pain control in advanced malignant disease using transcutaneous nerve stimulation. *B. J. Clin. Prac.*, **33**, 157–162.

Portenoy, R.K. (1989) Cancer pain: epidemiology and syndromes. *Cancer*, **63**, 2298–2307.

Rafter, J. (1986) TENS and cancer pain. Paper read to the Acupuncture Foundation of Canada Congress on Acupuncture and Related Techniques. Toronto, Canada, November 19–36.

Thompson, J.W. and Filshie J. (1998) Transcutaneous electrical nerve stimulation (TENS) and acupuncture, in *Oxford Textbook of Palliative Medicine*, 2nd edn (eds D. Doyle, G.W.C. Hanks and N. MacDonald), pp. 427–437, Oxford University Press, Oxford.

Part Two:
Rheumatic Pain

Painful joint: pathophysiology and treatment

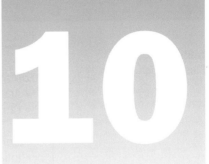

Patients presenting with pain constitute the bulk of a family physician's workload and this is also the most common complaint of patients presenting to a rheumatology clinic. The most common causes are osteoarthritis of the peripheral joints, back pain, strains and sprains, etc. The intensity of pain varies from mild pain requiring simple over-the-counter analgesia to severe pain requiring opioids. To identify the cause of the pain and to relieve the pain is the main concern of the patients and the physician treating the painful condition (Bombardier *et al.*, 1982).

The main function of a joint is movement and to maintain posture and balance. Pain in joints, however, is a very common condition which affects almost all of us sometime during our life. Painful joint, like pain anywhere else in the body, is a subjective, unpleasant feeling of varying intensity. Pain has been defined by the International Association for the Study of Pain as 'an unpleasant, sensory and emotional experience associated with actual or potential tissue damage or described in terms of such pain' (Merskey, 1986).

Function of pain

Pain is a body defence mechanism and protects the part involved, such as an inflamed or swollen joint, from further damage by limiting mobility. An inflamed painful joint therefore, when rested, usually promotes recovery by hastening tissue recovery. Pain also has a diagnostic value. The nature and character of pain, such as site, radiation, aggravating and relieving factors, are often helpful in identifying the cause of the pain.

Classification of pain

There are various ways in which pain can be classified (Table 10.1). Pain can be classified according to its duration as acute or chronic. **Acute pain** is

Table 10.1

Classification of pain

Duration
- Acute
- Chronic (pain of at least three months' duration)

Painful joint
- Inflammatory (rheumatoid arthritis)
- Mechanical or 'degenerative' (low back pain, osteoarthritis)

Pathophysiological classification
- Psychogenic (no idenitifiable organic cause)
- Organic
  Nociceptive (associated with potential or ongoing tissue damage)
  - (a) Superficial or cutaneous
  - (b) Deep or somatic (arthritic pain)
  - (c) Visceral (myocardial infarction)
  Neuropathic
  - (a) Central nervous system (thalamic syndrome)
  - (b) Peripheral nervous system (post-herpetic neuralgia)
- Mixed pain

---

usually associated with an obvious cause and commonly has an observed response, such as withdrawal of the painful joint due to acute sharp injury. Acute pain is accompanied by autonomic hyperactivity manifesting as anxiety, tachycardia, sweating and increased blood pressure. **Chronic pain** is defined as pain that persists for at least three months. Chronic pain can be persistent or intermittent and can be mild, moderate or severe. Patients with chronic pain adapt to the sympathetic overactivity and may not have the same physiological responses as found in acute pain. Examples of chronic pain include malignant pain associated with cancer and chronic non-malignant pain such as rheumatoid arthritis and low back pain.

Pain can be classified pathophysiologically as organic or psychological. In organic pain there is usually an identifiable cause. Organic pain can be nociceptive or neuropathic. Nociceptive pain is due to potential or ongoing tissue damage in response to a chemical, mechanical or noxious thermal stimulus. Nociceptive pain is further classified as superficial or cutaneous pain, deep or somatic pain, e.g. arthritic pain or bone pain of metastatic cancer, and visceral pain, which is poorly localized, deep in nature and may be referred, e.g. pain of cholecystitis or myocardial infarction.

Neuropathic pain arises from an abnormal or damaged nervous system without peripheral pain receptor stimulation. It is usually burning in character but can also be sharp and shooting. Neuropathic pain may also be experienced as paresthesias (electric shock type sensation), allodynia (abnormal sensation to light touch), dyesthesias (altered sensation) or hyperalgesia (extreme sensitivity to a mildly painful stimulus). It can be due to peripheral or central nervous system involvement. Examples include postherpetic neuralgia, thalamic syndrome, tumour infiltration of nerves and diabetic neuropathy.

Psychogenic pain or idiopathic pain has no organic cause. It has also been described as a somatoform pain disorder, which is a diagnosis of exclusion (American Psychiatric Association, 1994). Examples include pain during conversion hysteria and schizophrenic hallucinations.

Pain emanating from a joint can be classified as inflammatory pain, such as in rheumatoid arthritis, or degenerative pain which arises because of the mechanical derangement and destruction of the joint, such as in an osteoarthritic knee. Chronic pain is often mixed in origin, with psychological factors such fear and anxiety complicating the management of a nociceptive or neuropathic pain.

Anatomy of a joint

A typical joint consists of two bony articulating surfaces lined by hyaline cartilage. The articulating bones are held together by a capsule which is lined by synovium. The joint capsule is strengthened by ligaments and surrounding muscle.

Blood vessels and nerve supply

The synovial joint has a good blood supply and receives its nutrients mostly by diffusion. Hyaline cartilage lacks blood vessels and has no nerve supply. The synovium, however, has good arterial, venous and lymphatic systems extensively anastomosing with adjacent vessels of the capsule. The synovium generally is considered insensitive to pain; however, there is some evidence that it has isolated areas of sensory nerve fibres capable of transmitting pain (Kellgren and Samuel, 1950; Devillier et al., 1986).

The structures supporting the joint, i.e. the joint capsule, intra-articular fat pads, ligaments, periosteum and adjacent bone and muscles, however, are extensively innervated with receptors mainly for proprioception, but also for pain. Since the prime function of the joint is movement and balance, not surprisingly the main bulk of joint receptors deal with proprioception. The pain receptors normally are inactive, but can be stimulated by various mechanisms, such as chemical or mechanical noxious stimuli.

The nerve supply to joints arises from various sources, including small branches of peripheral nerves passing adjacent to the joints and branches of the intramuscular nerves of the muscles crossing the joint capsule. Most of the articular nerves are very small and not visible to the naked eye and hence surgical denervation of these small nerves rarely achieves successful long-term pain relief.

Chemical mediators

Nociceptive receptors are stimulated by the release of various chemical substances from the damaged tissue (Helme, Gibson and Khali, 1990). The initial sharp, well-localized pain is mediated by unmyelinated A delta fibres, while the dull throbbing pain which is poorly localized and more unpleasant is mediated by slow myelinated C fibres. The persistent pain predominantly results from the release of chemical mediators, such as bradykinin, from an inflamed joint. Bradykinins are the most potent pain-producing substances which cause vasodilatation of the small vessels, hence increasing capillary permeability, and they also cause vasoconstriction in the larger vessels. The bradykinins trigger the release of histamine and prostaglandin, and cause excitation of many nerve endings.

The other chemical transmitters include prostaglandins and neuro-transmitters, including 5-HT antihistamine and acetylcholine. Substance P, which may act as a neural transmitter at pain receptor sites, including sites for joint pain, may be involved in the release of bradykinin in histamine.

Neural pathways: peripheral receptors, spinal cord and brain

The peripheral pain receptors generate signals which are carried by both the myelinated and unmyelinated nerve fibres to the dorsal horn of the spinal cord (Figure 10.1). Most of the afferent nociceptive nerves terminate in a network in the substantia gelatinosa of the dorsal horn of spinal cord (Figure 10.2). The inhibitory interneurons in the substantia gelatinosa may act as a 'gate', blocking the upward transmission of pain impulses, in what is known as the 'gate control theory'. The gate may be closed by persistent C nociceptive fibre activation, descending inhibitory control system and mechanoreceptor activity (Figure 10.3; Searle, 1996). The gate opens for upward transmission of pain by the nociceptive A delta fibres.

The spinal cord and brain interact in a complex neural system with ascending and descending pathways (Figure 10.4).

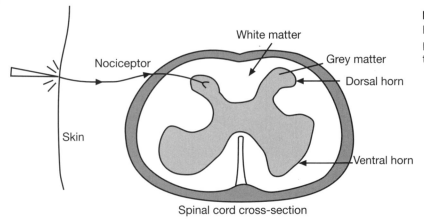

Figure 10.1
Neural transmission pathways: peripheral transmission.

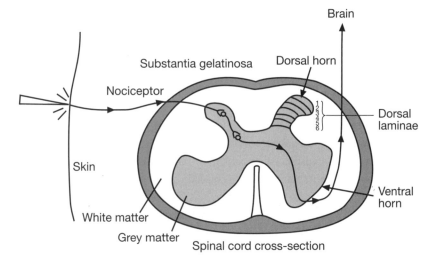

Figure 10.2
Neural transmission pathways: spinal cord transmission.
(Reprinted, with permission, from Searle, 1996.)

Intra-articular pressure

The normal resting intra-articular pressure is sub-atmospheric. The joint space usually has a small amount of fluid, even in a relatively large synovial joint such as the knee, hip or glenohumeral joint. The lax joint capsule usually helps in increased range of movement, such as in the glenohumeral joint. The lining of the joints is elastic and can be stretched by increasing the synovial fluid volume and hence increasing the intra-articular pressure. An increase in intra-articular pressure can lead to severe pain, particularly if it develops rapidly, such as in reactive or septic arthritis.

Figure 10.3
Gate control system for pain transmission: (a) acute pain; (b) persistent pain. (Reprinted, with permission, from Searle, 1996.)

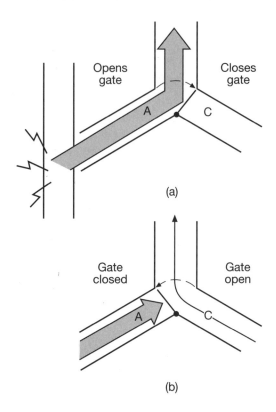

Pain due to an increase in intra-articular pressure is higher in a joint with a relatively tight capsule, such as the small joints of the fingers, toes or elbows, than in joints with a large synovial cavity, such as the glenohumeral or knee joint. When an effusion develops slowly, such as in a rheumatoid joint, pain may be less severe than an acutely inflamed or septic joint.

The increase in intra-articular pressure is also affected by the position of the joint. Weight bearing invariably increases pain in a swollen joint, owing to a further increase in intra-articular pressure.

Inflammatory versus mechanical pain

Although the aetiopathogenesis of rheumatoid arthritis and osteoarthritis are distinct and there are some differences between the nature of the pain produced by an inflammatory arthritis such as rheumatoid arthritis and pain produced by osteoarthritis, comparative studies of the two conditions have shown little difference in both the quality and quantity of joint pain (Bellamy and Buchanan, 1984; Charter, Nehemkis and Keenan, 1985).

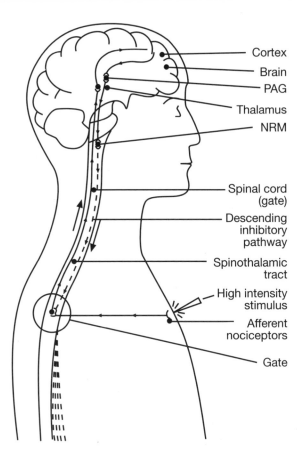

Cortex
Brain
PAG
Thalamus
NRM
Spinal cord
(gate)
Descending
inhibitory
pathway
Spinothalamic
tract
High intensity
stimulus
Afferent
nociceptors
Gate

Figure 10.4
Spinal cord–brain transmission. PAG, periaqueductal grey area; NRM, nucleus raphe magnus. (Reprinted, with permission, from Searle, 1996.)

The pain of osteoarthritis is usually produced by effort and relieved by rest, though a large proportion of patients with osteoarthritis also describe rest pain. The associated stiffness is less common in patients with osteoarthritis than in patients with an inflammatory arthritis. The pain of an inflamed joint during the early course of rheumatoid arthritis is predominantly produced by chemical mediators, unlike early osteoarthritis which can be asymptomatic. With the progression of osteoarthritis there is loss of cartilage and exposure of subchondral pain receptors, causing pain by rubbing the two denuded bony surfaces.

The pain arising from a chronic rheumatoid joint is predominantly due to a mixture of chemical and mechanical effects, while the pain of a burned out rheumatoid joint is purely mechanical and can be akin to an advanced osteoarthritic joint. The other contributing factors, such as raised intra-osseous pressure and pain arising from the elevation of the periosteum and from the stretching of the joint capsule, ligaments and surrounding muscles, contribute to pain in arthritis of both inflammatory and non-inflammatory origin.

Measurement of pain

Pain is a subjective feeling which is not easy to describe or measure, though there are various scales available to assess its severity, as described in Chapter 1.

The assessment of intensity of pain is particularly difficult in children or when there is a language or social barrier. There is still a lot of debate about the perception of pain by children, as some authors feel that children do not feel pain as much as adults. It is difficult to assess whether a child below the age of three experiences less pain or is not expressive enough to explain his or her feelings. Generally, however, the reporting of pain by those above the age of seven is comparable to that of the adult population.

The other end of the age group, i.e. elderly patients, also tend not to complain of pain and accept the painful joint as a part of the ageing process. Many elderly patients think that nothing more can be done if the first painkiller they take does not work. Pain management therefore should include not only a detailed patient evaluation, but also patient education and management at home.

Pharmacological treatment of pain in rheumatic diseases

Pain is the most common symptom of patients with rheumatic diseases such as rheumatoid arthritis, osteoarthritis and low back pain. The intensity of pain in rheumatic conditions usually varies from mild to moderate, but can be severe and debilitating.

The most important steps in pain management are:

- to identify the cause of the pain;
- to define the nature of the pain (acute or chronic, nociceptive, neurogenic or psychogenic);
- to begin appropriate analgesia;
- to educate the patient.

A detailed history, proper physical examination of the joints and relevant investigations will help in defining the pain and finding its cause. History and physical examination is often helpful in differentiating rheumatoid arthritis from osteoarthritis. Rheumatoid arthritis usually presents as a polyarthritis predominantly involving the small joints of the hands and feet, which are inflamed with soft tissue swelling, and the peak age of onset is between the third and fourth decades, while painful osteoarthritis predominantly affects the weight-bearing joints such as the knee, and the involved joint is enlarged predominantly due to hard bony swelling.

The choice of analgesia is dictated by the nature and severity of the pain and the experience of the prescriber in dealing with painful rheumatic diseases. Painful joints in an inflammatory arthritis such as rheumatoid arthritis also need second-line disease-modifying agents to prevent the progression, while treatment of a painful osteoarthritic knee is predominantly symptomatic.

Chronic pain of any cause and in particular pain associated with arthritis can be associated with fear and anxiety. Patient education should be included in the pharmacological and non-pharmacological management of pain. A proper explanation of the diagnosis, prognosis and treatment strategies available should be given to the patient in detail. Compliance is improved if the rationale of using a particular analgesic, such as the need for using the analgesia on an 'as required basis' or regular intake for 'around the clock' effect, is explained to patient.

The pharmacological agents commonly used for the treatment of rheumatic pain include:

- peripherally acting agents
- centrally acting agents
- adjuvant analgesic agents.

The World Health Organization has proposed a three-step analgesic ladder for the management of cancer pain (WHO, 1996). Its principle (Figure 10.5), however, can be applied to chronic pain of any cause, such as

Free from pain

Third step
Opioid for moderate to severe pain
Non-opioid
+Adjuvant

Pain persisting or increasing

Second step
Opioid for mild or moderate pain
Non-opioid
+Adjuvant

Pain resisting or increasing

First step
Non-opioid
+Adjuvant

Figure 10.5
World Health Organization three-step analgesic ladder.

chronic severe, painful arthritis. The first two steps are more relevant to rheumatic pain where initially the pain is treated with a non-opioid such as paracetamol or an NSAID followed by a weak opioid such as codeine or a compound preparation of paracetamol and dihydrocodeine.

NON-OPIOID AGENTS

These include the following agents which are very effective in mild to moderate pain.

Paracetamol

Paracetamol or acetaminophen is widely used and is very effective in mild to moderate pain of any cause. It inhibits the synthesis of prostaglandin synthetase in the central nervous system (Figure 10.6) but has virtually no inhibitory effect on the synthesis of peripheral prostaglandin (Rummans, 1994). Paracetamol does not appear to have any anti-inflammatory effect and therefore its role in the treatment of pain of inflammatory origin such

Figure 10.6
Mode of action of paracetamol. PAG, periaqueductal grey area; NRM, nucleus raphe magnus; LC, locus ceruleus. (Reprinted, with permission, from Searle, 1996.)

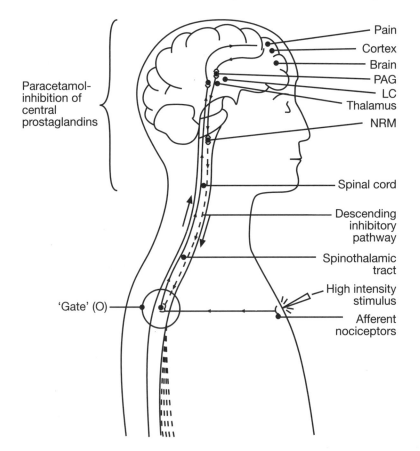

as rheumatoid arthritis is minimal. It is, however, very effective in non-inflammatory pain such as osteoarthritis and low back pain.

Non-steroidal anti-inflammatory drugs

Non-steroidal anti-inflammatory drugs (NSAIDs) are the most commonly prescribed drugs world wide and their use is increasing. There are already a large number of NSAIDs available in the market and in some countries some NSAIDs can be purchased over the counter. The number of NSAIDs available will increase further, with newer preparations offering prospects of less side-effects.

The NSAIDs are analgesic and anti-inflammatory. Their role in rheumatic conditions is purely symptomatic and they have no disease-modifying effect on conditions such as rheumatoid arthritis, for which they are most widely used. NSAIDs will give good symptomatic relief in an inflammatory arthritis, including juvenile arthritis. They are also helpful in spondyloarthropathies, psoriatic arthritis and reactive arthritis. NSAIDs are also widely used for low back and neck pain and for osteoarthritis. Their role should be limited in these conditions and it is better initially to try simple analgesia, such as paracetamol.

Rheumatic complaints are generally more common in the elderly, who are also more prone to the side-effects of NSAIDs, which should therefore be used with caution. It is better to familiarize oneself with one or two NSAIDs from different categories, such as those which are short acting (e.g. ibuprofen), intermediate (e.g. naproxen) and long acting (e.g. meloxicam) and those with a better relative safety profile, such as nabumetone, meloxicam and etodolac.

NSAIDs should not be used in combination as it is bound to increase the toxicity. It is important to warn patients that NSAIDs need to be taken regularly. A single dose of an NSAID has an analgesic effect perhaps comparable to paracetamol and does not have much anti-inflammatory action. With regular use the analgesic effect is stabilized within a week, while a significant anti-inflammatory effect may take up to 3 weeks.

Surprisingly the clinical response produced by different NSAIDs varies markedly among different individuals. A trial of a particular NSAID should be for at least 3–4 weeks before changing to another preparation. It is very common in patients with inflammatory arthritis to try three or four NSAIDs before a suitable one is identified.

Pharmacokinetics and mechanism of action

NSAIDs are commonly taken orally, though they can be administered in suppository or intramuscular form. They are also available in creams and gels, though the absorption from the skin is very poor (Figure 10.7).

Figure 10.7
Pharmacokinetics of NSAIDs.

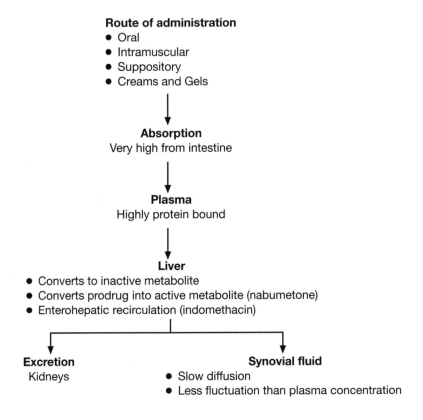

Route of administration
- Oral
- Intramuscular
- Suppository
- Creams and Gels

↓

Absorption
Very high from intestine

↓

Plasma
Highly protein bound

↓

Liver
- Converts to inactive metabolite
- Converts prodrug into active metabolite (nabumetone)
- Enterohepatic recirculation (indomethacin)

Excretion
Kidneys

Synovial fluid
- Slow diffusion
- Less fluctuation than plasma concentration

The absorption of an NSAID is very good from the gastrointestinal mucosa, almost all of it being absorbed. This absorption, however, is slowed if there is food in the stomach. Many non-steroidals are available in a slow-release or enteric-coated formulation so as to give a sustained release and hence stable plasma concentration.

Once in the circulation, NSAIDs are highly protein bound, the unbound concentration, i.e. the amount of free or active component, being relatively small. This fraction of NSAID tightly bound to albumin has a serious implication for drug interaction. Similarly any condition leading to hypoalbuminaemia will decrease the binding of an NSAID, thereby increasing the amount of free NSAID.

NSAIDs are distributed uniformly throughout the circulation. However, some such as ibuprofen, naproxen and ketoprofen are more lipid soluble and hence penetrate the central nervous system more easily.

Most of the NSAIDs are converted into inactive metabolites in the liver which are excreted in the urine. However, some of the NSAIDs such as nabumetone are converted into an active metabolite which is responsible for its pharmacological effect. While the majority of NSAIDs are excreted in the urine, some such as indomethacin also have enterohepatic recirculation, which may be responsible for increased gastric side-effects.

NSAIDs can be classified on the basis of their duration of action, i.e. plasma half-life. Some such as phenylbutazone, tenoxicam and piroxicam have a very long half-life compared to the short half-life of NSAIDs such as ibuprofen and tolmetin. Many of the short duration NSAIDs, however, are available in an enteric-coated or sustained-release formulation which gives them a longer half-life and a stable plasma concentration. It is, however, interesting that the fluctuation in the amount of an NSAID in the synovial fluid is much slower than its plasma concentration, even for the drugs with a relatively short plasma half-life.

NSAIDs belong to a variety of chemical classes with some differences in their pharmacokinetics resulting in differences in their mechanism of action and adverse reactions. The cellular mechanisms of action of NSAIDs are diverse and influence the synthesis of many chemicals, including prostaglandin (Figure 10.8), leukotriene, cytokine and nitric oxide.

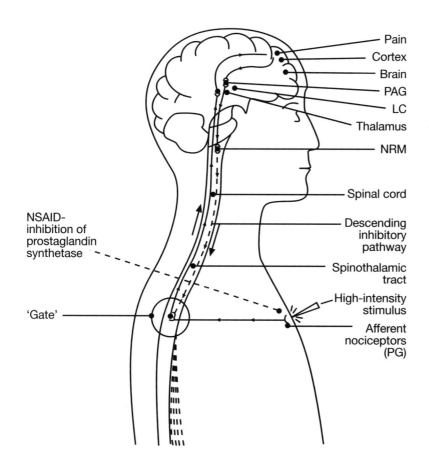

Figure 10.8
Mode of action of NSAIDs. PAG, periaqueductal grey area; NRM, nucleus raphe magnus; LC, locus ceruleus. (Reprinted, with permission, from Searle, 1996.)

It is widely accepted that many of the clinically beneficial as well as toxic effects of NSAIDs are due to inhibition of the synthesis of prostaglandins and thromboxanes. The traditional principal mechanism of action of NSAIDs has been recognized over the years as the inhibition of the enzyme cyclo-oxygenase (Cox). Recently, Cox has been shown to have two distinct isoenzymes, i.e. Cox-1 and Cox-2. The Cox-1 enzyme is called the 'house keeping' enzyme, as its main physiological actions appear to be the protection of the gastric mucosa, regulation of renal blood flow and platelet aggregation. The Cox-2 enzyme, on the other hand, reduces inflammation.

Most of the currently available NSAIDs inhibit both Cox-1 and Cox-2, though new compounds are undergoing clinical trials and early reports of short-term studies of very selective Cox-2 inhibitors are encouraging. These newer compounds have a very high selectivity for Cox-2 inhibition of 300-fold or more than that for Cox-1, compared to the currently available relatively Cox-2 selective NSAIDs where the inhibition of Cox-2 is 3–10-fold over Cox-1. They include meloxicam, nabumetone and etodolac.

Salicylates

Salicylates are also classified as NSAIDs. Those such as acetylsalicylic acid (aspirin) have both analgesic and anti-inflammatory effects, depending on the dose. Salicylates are rapidly absorbed and effective as an analgesic for mild to moderate pain.

CENTRALLY ACTING ANALGESICS

Opioids and tramadol hydrochloride are centrally acting analgesics widely used for pain control. These compounds are predominantly administered for moderate to severe acute and chronic pain. Their role in inflammatory pain is limited and they should be used sparingly in patients with arthritis of inflammatory or non-inflammatory origin. In the WHO analgesic ladder these compounds are included in the second step (Figure 10.5).

Opioid analgesics

Opioid analgesics are widely used and are very effective for pain relief. Table 10.2 gives the most commonly prescribed opioids. The opioids bind to specific opioid receptors in the brain and dorsal horn of the spinal cord (Figure 10.9). There are at least five different opioids receptors. Analgesia is produced by activation of the μ-, κ- and δ-receptors. These receptors are stimulated by endogenous peptides released by the stimulation of nociceptive receptors.

Opioid	Category	Alternative
Codeine	Weak opioid	Dihydrocodeine hydrochloride Dextropropoxyphene Tramadol
Morphine	Strong opioid	Pethidine Methadone Buprenorphine

Table 10.2
Commonly prescribed opioid analgesics

Some opioids (e.g. codeine) are relatively weak at producing analgesia compared to stronger opioids (e.g. morphine). This is due to a variation in binding to receptors by different opioids. Analgesia produced by the opioids is based on their action on specific receptors and accordingly opioids can be classified into various categories (Table 10.3).

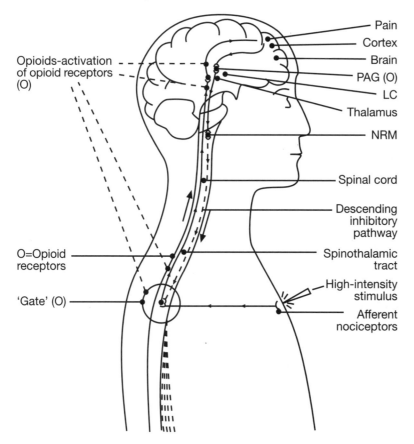

Figure 10.9
Mode of action of opioids. PAG, periaqueductal grey area; NRM, nucleus raphe magnus; LC, locus ceruleus. (Reprinted, with permission, from Searle, 1996.)

Table 10.3
Opioid classification

Receptor class	Action	Example
Agonist	Maximum receptor stimulation	Morphine
Partial agonist	Stimulates receptor below the maximum level	Buprenorphine
Mixed agonist–antagonist	Simultaneously acts on different receptor subtypes	Pentazocine

A true agonist such as morphine maximally stimulates the receptors and hence is a stronger analgesic. A true agonist has a straight dose–response curve, i.e. the analgesic effect increases in proportion to the increase in dose of the drug. A partial agonist such as buprenorphine, on the other hand, submaximally stimulates the opioid receptors and has a lesser effect than a pure agonist. The dose–response curve in a partial agonist tends to reach a plateau at a much lower rate. The third category of opioids is a mixed opioid, i.e. an agonist–antagonist such as pentazocine. These act simultaneously on different receptor subtypes. The fourth category is a pure antagonist such as naloxone which has no analgesic effect but is used to reverse the effects of opioid receptor stimulating drugs.

A combination of different categories of opioid receptor stimulating drugs, such as an agonist and partial agonist or agonist–antagonist, should not be used because it could lead to a reversal of the analgesic effect of a pure agonist in patients on a regular agonist analgesic.

The choice of an opioid analgesic depends on many factors, including its duration of action, efficacy, tolerance, side-effect profile and cost. The use of stronger opioids is limited in patients with rheumatic disease. These should not be used on a regular basis in patients with painful joints. There is a place for short-term use of opioids during the early days of a painful vertebral crush fracture and in patients with septic arthritis.

Tramadol

Tramadol is a synthetic centrally acting analgesic with a dual mode of action (Figure 10.10). It acts predominantly at central μ opiate receptors and also inhibits the re-uptake of serotonin and norepinephrine. It is well absorbed from the gastrointestinal mucosa and has no upper gastrointestinal side-effects such as ulceration or bleeding (Taniguchi and Icaza, 1997). It has a very minimal effect on colonic transit but no effect on the upper gastrointestinal transit or gut smooth muscle tone (Wilder-Smith and Bettiga, 1997). Tramadol is metabolized in the liver. Its analgesic effect begins

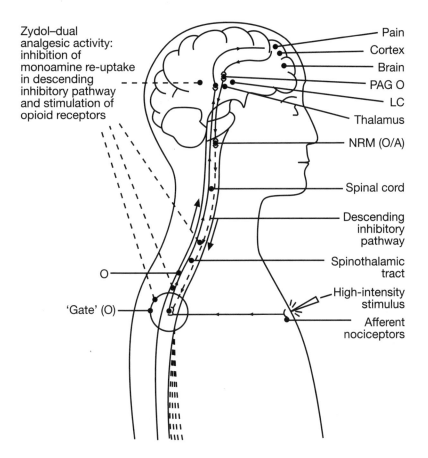

Zydol–dual analgesic activity: inhibition of monoamine re-uptake in descending inhibitory pathway and stimulation of opioid receptors

Pain
Cortex
Brain
PAG O
LC
Thalamus
NRM (O/A)
Spinal cord
Descending inhibitory pathway
Spinothalamic tract
High-intensity stimulus
Afferent nociceptors
O
'Gate' (O)

Figure 10.10
Mode of action of tramadol. PAG, periaqueductal grey area; NRM, nucleus raphe magnus; LC, locus ceruleus. (Reprinted, with permission, from Searle, 1996.)

within one hour. It has been reported to have less opioid side-effects, such as respiratory depression, constipation and low potential for abuse or addiction (Taniguchi and Icaza, 1997). Tramadol is available in oral, intravenous and intramuscular preparations. The usual oral dose is 50–100 mg every 4–6 hours (Katz, 1996).

Tramadol is effective for moderate to severe pain (Gibson, 1996). Its analgesic efficacy lies between that of codeine and morphine. In the WHO three-steps analgesic ladder (Figure 10.5) tramadol should be considered an alternative in step 2.

The use of tramadol in patients with rheumatic disease is well established. Tramadol is an analgesic and has no disease-modifying effect on inflammatory arthritis such as rheumatoid arthritis. Its therapeutic indications are in pain of moderate to severe intensity, such as acute severe low back pain not responding to simple analgesia, pain in vertebral crush fractures, and the severe pain of septic arthritis. Tramadol is also effective for chronic pain relief in osteoarthritis of the hips and knee (Katz, 1996), rheumatoid arthritis (Vlak, 1996) and for chronic moderate to severe low back pain. For patients with chronic pain, a slow-release formulation may be appropriate.

Tramadol is also effective for moderate to severe cancer pain (Wilder-Smith *et al.*, 1994; Bono and Cuffari, 1997; Taniguchi and Icaza, 1997). In one study it was found to be more effective than buprenorphine in tumour pain (Brema *et al.*, 1996). Tramadol has also been found to be a good analgesic in postherpetic pain (Gobel and Stadler, 1997), acute post-operative pain (Lehmann, 1997), dento-alveolar pain (Collins *et al.*, 1997) and labour pain (Taniguchi and Icaza, 1997).

Compound analgesics

Different combinations of weak opioids such as codeine, dihydrocodeine and dextropropoxyphene with paracetamol or aspirin are widely available. The logic of prescribing a compound analgesia is to have a dual analgesic effect, i.e. peripherally with paracetamol and centrally with an opioid (Figure 10.11). Table 10.4 gives a list of analgesic preparations commonly prescribed in the UK.

Figure 10.11
Mode of action of compound analgesics. PAG, periaqueductal grey area; NRM, nucleus raphe magnus; LC, locus ceruleus. (Reprinted, with permission, from Searle, 1996.)

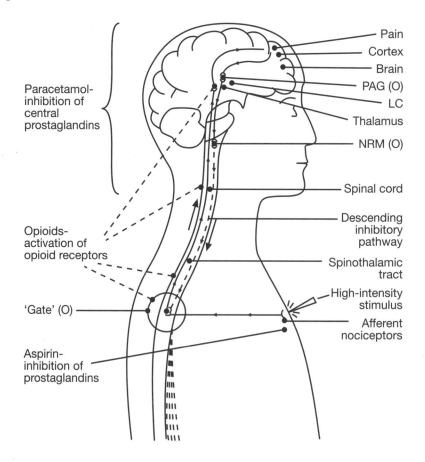

Compound analgesics are mostly used for mild to moderate pain when the pain relief is not adequately achieved by a simple analgesic such as aspirin, paracetamol or an NSAID. Compound analgesics carrying a full dose of an opioid can cause the usual side-effects, including nausea, vomiting, constipation, drowsiness, respiratory depression and addiction, and therefore should be used with caution particularly in the elderly and those with hepatic and renal impairment. These compounds are dangerous in overdose.

Table 10.4

Compound preparations of aspirin, paracetamol, opioids and NSAIDs

Compound preparations with aspirin	
Name (proprietary)	**Constituents**
Co-codaparin	aspirin 400 mg, codeine 8 mg
Doloxene compound	aspirin 375 mg, dextropropoxyphene hydrochloride and caffeine 30 mg
Aspav	aspirin 500 mg, morphine hydrochloride 5 mg, papaverine hydrochloride 600 µg, codeine hydrochloride 520 µg

Compound preparations with paracetamol	
Name (proprietary)	**Constituents**
Co-codamol	paracetamol 500 mg, codeine phosphate 8 mg
Solpadol	paracetamol 500 mg, codeine phosphate 30 mg
Tylex	paracetamol 500 mg, codeine phosphate 30 mg
Co-dydramol	paracetamol 500 mg, dihydrocodeine tartarate 10 mg
Co-proxamol	paracetamol 350 mg, dextropropoxyphene hydrochloride 32.5 mg
Fortagesic	paracetamol 500 mg, pentazocine hydrochloride 15 mg
Pradote	paracetamol 500 mg, co-methiamol 100 mg

Compound preparations with NSAIDs	
Name (proprietary)	**Constituents**
Codafen Continus	Ibuprofen 300 mg, codeine phosphate 20 mg

Other compound proprietary preparations containing ibuprofen include Neurofen Plus and Solpaflex

ADJUVANT ANALGESIC AGENTS

Chronic persistent pain very frequently leads to interrupted sleep, irritability and depression. Patients with chronic persistent pain may benefit from a small dose of an antidepressant such as a tricyclic antidepressant. Antidepressants may improve both the depression and the pain, or only the depression and have no effect on the pain. A small proportion of patients with chronic pain and no apparent depression may achieve benefit in pain, suggesting an analgesic effect independent of antidepressant activity.

Tricyclic antidepressants can be effective in painful conditions such as fibromyalgia, chronic low back and neck pain, and in neuropathic pain (Magni, 1991). The analgesic effect of a regular low dose antidepressant may occur within 4–7 days of initiating therapy, whereas the antidepressant activity usually occur after 3–4 weeks.

The main mechanism of action in the treatment of chronic pain appears to be due to the enhancement of the endogenous pain-inhibiting system (Saatterthwaite, Tollison and Kriegel, 1990). Norepinephrine and serotonin are important neurotransmitters and their re-uptake at the synapses appears to be inhibited by tricyclic antidepressants, thereby facilitating central monoaminergic transmission (Garcia and Altman, 1997).

The analgesic efficacy of second generation antidepressants such as paroxetine and fluoxetine has not been adequately assessed and therefore should not be used instead of tricyclic antidepressants for the treatment of pain. The most commonly prescribed tricyclic antidepressant is amitriptyline, which should be used at a dose of 10–30 mg at night. The other commonly used tricyclic antidepressants include dothiepin hydrochloride, doxepin, clomipramine and imipramine. Tricyclic antidepressants should be discontinued if there is no clinical improvement after 4–6 weeks of treatment.

Anticonvulsants such as carbamazepine and phenytoin and benzodiazepines such as diazepam and lorazepam have been used in the management of chronic neuropathic pain (Chernyl and Protenoy, 1994), but these generally are of no benefit in painful rheumatic conditions. Intravenous infusions of local anaesthetics such as lignocaine (Boas, Conino and Sahnorian, 1982) and mexiletine have been reported to give pain relief lasting for hours to days. These drugs perhaps have some limited role in the management of chronic diffuse pain. There are, however, no well-controlled comparative studies available to recommend their use in painful rheumatic conditions.

References

American Psychiatric Association (1994) *Diagnostic and Statistical Manual of Mental Disorders*, 4th edn, American Psychiatric Association, Washington, DC.

Bellamy, N. and Buchanan W.W. (1984) Outcome measurement in osteoarthritis clinical trials: the case of standardization. *Clin. Rheumatol.*, **3**, 293–303.

Boas, R.A., Conino, B.G, and Sahnorian, A. (1982) Analgesic response to IV lignocaine. *Br. J. Anaesth.*, **54**, 501–504.

Bombardier, C., Tugwell B., Sinclair A., *et al.* (1982) Preference for end point measure in clinical trials; results of structured workshops. *J. Rheumatol.*, **9**, 798–801.

Bono, A.V. and Cuffari S. (1997) Effectiveness and tolerance of tramadol in cancer pain. A comparative study with respect to buprenorphine [in French]. *Drugs*, **53**, Suppl. 2, 40–49.

Brema F., Pastorino G., Martini, M.C. *et al.* (1996) Oral tramadol and buprenorphine in tumour pain. An Italian multicentre trial. *Int. J. Clin. Pharm. Res.*, **16**(4–5), 109–116.

Charter, R.A., Nehemkis, A.M. and Keenan, M.A. (1985) The nature of arthritis pain. *Br. J. Rheumatol.*, **24**, 53–60.

Chernyl, N.I. and Protenoy R.K. (1994) The management of cancer pain. *Cancer J. Clin.*, **44**, 262–303.

Collins, M., Young I., Sweeney P. *et al.* (1997) The effect of tramadol on dento-alveolar surgical pain. *Br. J. Oral Maxillofacial Surg.*, **35**(1), 54–58.

Devillier, P., Weill B., Renoux, M. *et al.* (1986) Elevated levels of tachykinin like immuno-reactivity in joint fluids from patients. *N. Eng. J. Med.*, **314**, 1323–1330.

Garcia, J. and Altman, R.D. (1997) Chronic pain states: pathophysiology and medical therapy. *Semin. Arth. Rheum.*, **27**,(1), 1–16.

Gibson, T.P. (1996) Pharmacokinetics, efficacy, and safety of analgesia with a focus on tramadol HCL. *Am. J. Med.*, **101**(1A), 47S–53S.

Gobel, H. and Stadler, T. (1997) Treatment of post-herpes zoster pain with tramadol. Results of an open pilot study versus clomipramine with or without levomepromazine [in French]. *Drugs*, **53**, Suppl. 2, 34–39.

Helme, R.D., Gibson, S. and Khalil, Z. (1990) Neural pathways in chronic pain. *Med. J. Aust.*, **153**, 400–409.

Katz, W.A. (1996) Pharmacology and clinical experience with tramadol in osteoarthritis. *Drugs*, **52**, Suppl. 3, 39–47.

Kellgren, J.H. and Samuel E.P. (1950) The sensitivity and innovation of the articular capsule. *J. Bone Joint Surg.*, **32b**, 84–92.

Lehmann, K.A. (1997) Tramadol in acute pain [in French]. *Drugs*, **53**, Suppl. 2, 25–33.

Levick, J.R. (1979) An investigation into the validity of subatmospheric pressure recordings from synovial fluid and their dependence on joint angle. *J. Physiol.*, **289**, 55–67.

Magni, G. (1991) The use of anti-depressants in the treatment of chronic pain. *Drugs*, **42**, 730–748.

Merskey, H.M. (1986) Classification of chronic pain syndrome [Abstract]. *Pain*, Suppl. 3, S217.

Rummans, T.A. (1994) Nonopioid agents for treatment of acute and subacute pain. *Mayo Clin. Proc.*, **69**, 481–490.

Saatterthwaite J.R., Tollison C.D. and Kriegel M.L. (1990) The use of tricyclic antidepressants in the treatment of chronic intractable pain. *Compr. Ther.*, **16**, 10–15.

Searle (1996) *Pain exchange; current thinking on pain relief.* ZY: ATW 596.

Taniguchi, G. and Icaza, I. (1997) Criteria for use of tramadol hydrochloride in adult inpatients and outpatients. *Am. J. Health-System Pharm.*, **54**(6), 696–697.

Vlak, T. (1996) Tramadol (Tramal) in the treatment of rheumatic diseases – comparative study [Serbo-Croation study]. *Rheumatizm*, **43**(2), 1–10.

Wilder-Smith, C.H. and Bettiga, A. (1997) The analgesic tramadol has minimal effect on gastrointestinal motor function. *Brit. J. Clin. Pharmacol.*, **43**(1), 71–75.

Wilder-Smith, C.H., Schimke J., Osterwalder, B. *et al.* (1994) Oral tramadol, a mu-opioid agonist and monoamine reuptake-blocker, and morphine for strong cancer-related pain. *Ann. Oncol.*, **5**(2), 141–146.

WHO (1996) *Cancer pain relief and palliative care: report of a WHO expert committee*, 2nd edn. World Health Organization, Geneva.

Rheumatoid arthritis

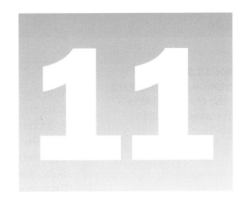

Rheumatoid arthritis is the commonest and one of the most severe forms of inflammatory polyarthritis. In historical terms rheumatoid arthritis is a relatively new entity. It was Garrod (Garrod, 1859) who in 1859 coined the term rheumatoid arthritis, though there is convincing evidence from both the medical and non-medical literature as to the existence of this disease before the first accepted description of it in the early 1800s by Landre-Beaubais (Snorrason, 1952).

Epidemiology

Rheumatoid arthritis is the commonest inflammatory polyarthritis and it has been found in almost all ethnic groups that have been studied so far. It is two to three times more common in women. However, the prevalence increases with age in both sexes. There appears to be a difference in its prevalence among different ethnic groups. The highest reported prevalence so far has been reported in the Pima Indians of Arizona (5.3%) and the Chippewa of Minnesota (also 5.3%). The prevalence in Caucasians is about 1% and in the Oriental population 0.3–0.6%. Its prevalence in the Asian and African adult population is also quite low.

There appears to be high mortality in rheumatoid arthritis compared to age- and sex-matched individuals from the general population (Symmons, 1988; Myllkangas-Luosujarvi, Aho and Isomaki, 1995a; Symmond, 1995), though causes of death appear to be the same as in the general population (Symmons, 1988). The excess mortality in rheumatoid arthritis has been attributed to the disease itself as well as to the drugs used in its management (Myllkangas-Luosujarvi, Ako and Isomaki, 1995b).

There is a strong association of rheumatoid arthritis with HLA DR 4. The subtype Dw14 is more strongly associated with rheumatoid arthritis in Caucasians (Nepom, Hansen and Nepom, 1987) while DR1 is more strongly associated with rheumatoid arthritis in Asian Indians, Hispanics and Israeli Jews (Smith and Arnett, 1991).

Table 11.1
Revised diagnostic criteria for the classification of rheumatoid arthritis (1987)

Morning stiffness of at least one hour[a]
Arthritis in at least three joint areas[b] with swelling or fluid[a]
Arthritis of hand joints (at least one area swollen in a wrist, MCP, or PIP joint)[a]
Symmetrical joint swelling and involvement[a]
Subcutaneous nodules
Radiographic changes typical of RA
Positive rheumatoid factor

[a] specified criteria that must be present for at least six weeks
[b] right or left proximal interphalangeal (PIP), metacarpophalangeal (MCP), wrist, elbow, knee, ankle and metatarsophalangeal (MTP) joint.

The American Rheumatism Association criteria of 1987 are widely used for the classification of rheumatoid arthritis (Table 11.1). These criteria were initially developed in 1956 and revised in 1958, then further modified and made simpler in 1987.

Clinical features

Rheumatoid arthritis is a multisystem disorder in which joint involvement is the main feature. In most cases the onset of rheumatoid arthritis is gradual. However, it can also present in sub-acute form or with an abrupt onset (Fleming, Crown and Corbett, 1976).

The commonest presentation of rheumatoid arthritis is predominantly articular, affecting the small joints of the hands and feet, with systemic features of generalized aches and pains and morning stiffness of variable duration. Rheumatoid arthritis can also commence as a monoarthritis, though this presentation is less common.

The natural course of rheumatoid arthritis consists of remissions and exacerbations. In most cases, rheumatoid arthritis leads to progressive joint damage resulting in significant pain and physical disabilities. With the passage of time the rheumatoid arthritis can 'burn' itself out. Patients in which this has occurred have pain predominantly secondary to degenerative changes in the joints rather than pain of inflammatory arthritis.

The bad prognostic factors in rheumatoid arthritis include acute onset, positive rheumatoid factor, male sex and those with early radiological changes. Female sex hormones have an important influence on rheumatoid arthritis. Rheumatoid arthritis improves in about 70% of women during pregnancy (Nicholas and Panayi, 1988). The role of sex hormones is further indicated by some other studies, which showed a decreased incidence of rheumatoid arthritis in women with previous pregnancies, those taking oral contraceptives and post-menopausal women on oestrogen-replacement therapy (Carette, Marcoux and Gingras, 1989; Hazas *et al.*, 1990; Spector *et al.*, 1991). Recent studies have reported a falling incidence of rheumatoid arthritis in women (Linos *et al.*, 1980; Wicks, Moore and Fleming, 1988), the exact cause of which is unknown.

Management

Pain is the cardinal feature of inflammation. The exact cause of localized inflammation in rheumatoid arthritis is unknown. It is, however, accepted that some unknown antigen is presented by the macrophages to the inflammatory cells. These cells then release inflammatory markers, including cytokines and interleukins. These inflammatory markers are responsible for proliferation of the synovial cells, which further release inflammatory markers and cause pannus formation. The inflammatory cytokines released at the joint act locally as well as systemically.

Inflammatory pain involving articular and periarticular areas is the most disabling symptom during the early course. It occurs at rest as well as on movement, and can be localized to one joint, though usually it originates from multiple sites.

The management of pain relief for an inflamed joint consists of:

- non-Pharmacological therapy
- pharmacological therapy.

Non-pharmacological therapy for rheumatoid arthritis

Non-pharmacological agents include heat, cold, hydrotherapy and other physical therapy modalities. Non-pharmacological therapies have been used successively over hundreds of years to reduce pain and swelling. However, their exact mode of action remains unknown.

HEAT

Superficial, deep and moist or dry heat has been widely used for pain relief of an inflamed joint. Superficial heat is mainly administered in the form of hot packs, hot water, paraffin and convective fluidotherapy, while deep heat with the use of ultrasound or short-wave and microwave diathermy can elevate the temperature of tissue up to 5 cm or more beneath the skin surface.

Heat reduces local pain and muscle spasm. This local effect of heat obviously depends on the amount of energy delivered and the surface area treated. The local application of heat can decrease joint stiffness (Backlund and Tiselius, 1967) and direct application of heat can increase the extensibility of the collagen tissue (Leban, 1962; Warren, Lehmann and Koblanski, 1976).

Cold

Cold has an analgesic action presumably through its effect in decreasing the sensitivity of the muscle spindle afferent discharge. It decreases oedema through cutaneous vasoconstriction, hence decreasing blood flow, which can decrease local inflammation. There is evidence that superficial application of cold may reduce joint blood flow in an animal model (Ekblom *et al.*, 1974). It has also been reported that the local application of cold improves the range of motion in frozen shoulder (Danneskiold-Samsoe and Grimby, 1986) as well as pain and sleep in patients with knee pain (Nordesjo, Nordgren and Wigren, 1983).

Local cold for an inflamed joint or periarticular area can be applied in the form of cold packs, ice cubes or bags of frozen pellets or even peas (Barls *et al.*, 1985). Local cold therapy should be applied with caution in patients with Raynaud's or other vascular pathology (Banwell, 1986).

There is wide variation about the time required for the local application of the cold. It depends on the individual's sensitivity as well as on the amount of his or her subcutaneous fat. In a thin person it may take only 5–10 minutes, while an obese person may require up to 30 minutes.

There is lack of data as to the advantage over using cold over heat for the treatment of inflammatory arthritis and the decision is often based on personal experience and the availability of treatment. However, since deep heat can increase the rate of collagen breakdown by specific enzymes, there is a theoretical possibility of increasing joint destruction by deep-heat treatment (Feibel and Fast, 1976). The general recommendations are to apply superficial heat for soft-tissue problems and mechanical arthritis, such as osteoarthritis, and to avoid using heat in an inflamed joint, where cold therapy is usually more helpful.

The other non-pharmacological modalities in the treatment of rheumatoid arthritis include hydrotherapy, acupuncture and transcutaneous electrical nerve stimulation.

Rheumatoid arthritis is a chronic disabling condition and it is therefore very important to have a team approach to its management. The role of the physiotherapist, occupational therapist and rheumatology practice nurse, who has a clear understanding of the condition and its treatment, plays an important part in the management of rheumatoid arthritis.

Drug treatment of pain in rheumatoid arthritis

This includes:

- simple analgesics and non-steroidal anti-inflammatory drugs;
- second-line disease-modifying agent;
- aspiration and intra-articular cortisone injection.

Rheumatoid arthritis is a complex multisystem disorder, but as far as the patient is concerned pain is the major disabling factor, particularly in the early stages of the disease. The pain due to inflammatory arthritis is present most of the time, but is worse during the morning, with marked stiffness in the joints.

The pharmacological approach to the management of rheumatoid arthritis has traditionally been in the form of a pyramid, with initial treatment with non-steroidal anti-inflammatory drugs (NSAIDs) followed by the addition of a disease-modifying agent and cytotoxic agent with or without regular use of steroids. Since joint damage starts very early in the course of rheumatoid arthritis, the pyramid approach has been replaced by more aggressive therapy during the early course of the disease.

Generally the majority of patients with rheumatoid arthritis are initially treated with one or the other form of a non-steroidal anti-inflammatory drug. Those with very mild inflammatory synovitis and those with palindromic arthritis of short duration get good symptomatic control from a non-steroidal anti-inflammatory drug. However, as the disease progresses and becomes more widespread, it is usually difficult to control the activity with an NSAID only and patients require additional treatment with a second-line disease-modifying agent. In addition, some patients require the use of corticosteroids for a variable period.

NON-STEROIDAL ANTI-INFLAMMATORY DRUGS

During the last century and during the major part of this century, aspirin was widely used as an antipyretic and anti-inflammatory agent with good results. However, during the past two to three decades there has been a widespread interest in NSAIDs, resulting in an enormous increase in their number. NSAIDs are one of the commonest drugs prescribed by general practitioners in the UK for a variety of rheumatological conditions.

Indications in rheumatoid arthritis

Non-steroidal anti-inflammatory drugs belong to a variety of chemical classes with slightly different mode, duration of action and toxicity. They can be classified according to their duration of action as short acting, long acting or medium acting, or as slow release or modified formulation (Table 11.2).

Almost all patients with rheumatoid arthritis are given NSAIDs in one form or another during the course of their disease. NSAIDs give symptomatic relief of pain and swelling, and hence improve the well-being of the patient. There is, however no evidence that these drugs have a disease-modifying effect (McConkey et al., 1973) and therefore they are unlikely to prevent progressive joint damage.

There are over 30 different NSAID preparations on the market in the UK. The choice usually is dictated by personal experience, but other factors such as patient's age, dosing regimen, efficacy and cost also play a major part. Caution should be exercised in selecting an NSAID particularly in patients with a previous history of peptic ulcers and those with renal impairment, especially in the elderly.

During early rheumatoid arthritis most of these patients are treated only with an NSAID, but as the disease becomes established a second-line disease-modifying agent is added to the treatment. Patients with rheumatoid arthritis generally need a more potent NSAID at a relatively high dose when they are not on a disease-modifying agent, but once the disease activity is controlled with the addition of a disease-modifying agent or a corticosteroid it is prudent to switch these patients to a less potent NSAID. Not all the NSAIDs work in every patient with rheumatoid arthritis and it is therefore recommended that an NSAID be changed to another preparation if there is no significant improvement after 2–3 weeks of regular use at full dose.

Table 11.2
Half-life of NSAIDs

Short (< 6 hours)	Medium (6–18 hours)	Long (> 18 hours)
Aspirin	Februfen	Meloxicam
Diclofenac	Naproxen	Piroxicam
Ibuprofen	Diflunisal	Tenoxicam
Etodolac	Sulindac	Nabumetone
Indomethacin	Azapropazone	Phenylbutazone
Ketoprofen		

Because of the enhanced toxicity it is advisable not to use different types of NSAIDs at the same time.

Some patients prefer using short acting NSAIDs, i.e. ones that last for 3–4 hours, such as ibuprofen, while those with significant nocturnal symptoms and morning stiffness prefer a long acting preparation where the therapeutic effects last 8–12 hours (Table 11.2).

NSAIDs are also available in the form of gel, suppositories and intra-muscular injections. For significant inflammatory polyarthritis such as rheumatoid arthritis there is very limited use for topical applications. NSAIDs in the suppository form are as effective as when taken orally. However, their use is limited because the majority of patients in the UK do not like to use drugs in suppository form. Non-steroidal anti-inflammatory suppositories in children, however, are used quite commonly with good effect. The side-effect profile of NSAIDs drug used in suppository form is comparable to that of NSAIDs administered orally. Some NSAIDs are available in the intramuscular form. They are not, however, used regularly in the treatment of rheumatoid arthritis, though they can be used short term during rheumatoid arthritis flares.

As the disease progresses painful joints are predominantly due to degenerative changes, with a much smaller inflammatory component. At this stage the swelling in joints is mostly bony with no active synovitis and both clinically and biochemically there is no evidence of significant inflammatory changes. In this situation it is better to control the pain with the addition of a simple analgesic such as paracetamol or a small dose of codeine rather than to use an NSAID.

NSAIDs are potentially toxic and can cause dyspepsia, gastric or small bowel perforation and bleeding. Other common-side effects include rashes and renal and hepatic impairment.

All NSAIDs can cause severe gastric side-effects and therefore should be used with caution, particularly in those at risk, i.e. those with a previous history of peptic ulcers or bleed, in the elderly and when used concomitantly with corticosteroids. Some NSAIDs, because of their mechanism of action, have less gastric side-effects compared to the others. Nabumetone, etodolac and meloxicam give less inhibition of Cox-2, which theoretically should cause less damage to the gastric mucosa. However, even these NSAIDs can cause serious gastric side-effects and it is prudent to use some form of gastric protection in susceptible individuals. Gastric protection can be provided by an H_2 inhibitor, such as ranitidine, proton pump inhibitors, such as omeprazole, or a prostaglandin analogue, such as misoprostol. The gastric protection provided by these agents is not complete, but so far in clinical studies misoprostol has been shown to be protective at both the gastric and the duodenal sites. Misoprostol itself is not free from side-effects and hence its use is limited. The susceptible individuals requiring long-term NSAIDs should be prescribed some form of gastric protection. My own preference for the susceptible group is to use misoprostol in combination with an NSAID and to monitor the patient closely for dyspeptic symptoms.

DISEASE-MODIFYING AGENTS

These drugs are also called slow-acting antirheumatic drugs or second-line agents, as generally they are not used as a first line. There is convincing evidence that damage to the inflamed joints occurs quite early in the course of rheumatoid athritis, particularly in the first two years. The MRI scan in early rheumatoid arthritis has been reported as showing erosive changes when the plain X-rays were normal.

The use of second-line agents for the treatment of rheumatoid arthritis started in the early part of this century when rheumatoid arthritis was considered to have an infective aetiology. Gold has antibacterial activity and was also successfully used for the treatment of rheumatoid arthritis. Indeed, it is still used in the treatment of rheumatoid arthritis, although this use is declining.

The use of antimalarials for the treatment of rheumatoid arthritis came about largely by serendipity. Salazopyrin was the first drug specifically developed for rheumatoid arthritis and is still widely used as a single agent and in different combinations for its treatment. With the recognition that rheumatoid arthritis is an autoimmune condition, azathioprine and penicillamine were introduced as immunosuppresive agents. This was followed by cytotoxic therapy, including methotrexate and cyclophosphamide and more recently cyclosporin. Table 11.3 summarizes the disease-modifying agents currently used in the treatment of rheumatoid arthritis.

Since damage to joints occurs during the early course of rheumatoid arthritis, it makes clinical sense to prescribe these drugs early on. It is generally recommended to start a disease-modifying agent once a diagnosis is established. In the UK the majority of rheumatologists use salazopyrin as their first second-line agent. This is usually followed by methotrexate with or without salazopyrin. Some centres recommend early aggressive combination chemotherapy to prevent joint damage during the early course of the disease and the results of these studies are keenly awaited. The second-line agents can be used in different combinations, the most common of which are methotrexate/salazopyrin, methotrexate/hydroxychloroquine and gold/hydroxychloroquine.

Second-line disease-modifying agents are not primarily given for pain relief and patients with rheumatoid arthritis need to take an NSAID for

Drug	Dosage regimen	Approximate time to benefit (weeks)
Sulphasalazine	1000 mg bid or rarely tid	4–8
Hydroxychloroquine	200 mg bid	8–16
Gold		
oral	3 mg once or bid	16–24
injectable	25–50 mg IM every 2–4 weeks	12–24
Methotrexate	7.5–15 mg once a week	4–8
Azathioprine	50–150 mg daily	8–12
D-Penicillamine	250–750 mg daily	12–24
Cyclosporin	2.5–5 mg/kg/day	4–12
Cyclophosphamide	1.5 mg/kg/day	4–16

symptomatic control along with these agents. However, once there is a definite improvement in symptoms with regular use of disease-modifying agents, the use of NSAIDs can be decreased. The disease-modifying drugs take some time to act (Table 11.3) and patients should be warned accordingly. Sometimes it can take as long as 12–16 weeks to notice significant clinical improvement. Methotrexate, however, can give clinically significant improvement within 4 weeks.

The second-line disease-modifying agents are potentially toxic and have various side-effects (Table 11.4). Patients on disease-modifying agents require regular monitoring, for which there are various published guidelines (American College of Rheumatology Ad Hoc Committee on Guidelines, 1996).

GLUCORTICOIDS

Corticosteroids have been used since the beginning of this century for the treatment of rheumatoid arthritis. Owing to their various side-effects, the long-term use of oral corticosteroids has declined. They are, however, still used in short courses when the disease-modifying antirheumatic agents are initiated, as steroids minimize disease activity fairly quickly, while the disease-modifying antirheumatic agents usually take a few weeks. A short course, 1–2 weeks, of oral corticosteroids is also helpful during a flare up of rheumatoid arthritis. In some patients, particularly the elderly where polymyalgia rheumatica commonly coexists, a low daily dose of prednisolone (5–10 mg) is very effective. The low-dose steroid needs to be taken on a daily basis as alternate day therapy usually does not produce significant clinical improvement.

Despite the extensive use of corticosteroids in rheumatoid arthritis there is still a lack of large, well-controlled long-term studies. Therefore despite their extensive use, controversy persists as to the long-term use of these agents in rheumatoid arthritis.

A study published in 1995 (Kirwan, 1995) reported a reduction in joint erosions in rheumatoid arthritis patients treated with corticosteroids compared to placebo. There has been extensive review of this paper and many authors have raised concern about its recommendation. The issues raised include the unintentional skewing of patients with more severe erosive disease into the placebo group and a lack of a control for second-line drug treatment and low use of methotrexate in the study population. There has

Table 11.4
Monitoring guidelines for patients on disease-modifying agents

Drug	Potential toxicity	Laboratory monitoring	
Sulphasalazine	Myelosuppression	FBC and liver transaminases, G6PD in at-risk patients	FBC every 2–4 weeks for first 3 months, then every 3 months
Hydroxychloroquine	Macular damage	Fundoscopy and visual field assessment by an ophthalmologist	Fundoscopy and visual field assessment at 6-month intervals
Gold			
(a) oral	Myelosuppression, proteinuria	FBC including platelet count, serum creatinine and urine dipstick analysis for protein	(a) FBC including platelet count; urine dipstick analysis every 4–12 weeks
(b) injectable			(b) FBC including platelet count; urine dipstick analysis every 1–2 weeks for 20 weeks, then before each injection
Azathioprine	Myelosuppression, hepatotoxic, lymphoproliferative disorders	FBC, platelet count, creatinine, AST or ALT; high-risk patients hepatitis B and C serology	FBC, platelet count every 1–2 weeks when dose is changed, then 1–3 months afterwards
D-Penicillamine	Myelosuppression, proteinuria	FBC, platelet count, creatinine and urine dipstick analysis	FBC, urine dipstick every 2 weeks; once dose is stabilized, every 1–3 months

FBC, full blood count (haemoglobin, haematocrit, total white cell count with differential count including platelet); CXR, chest X-ray; AST, aspartate aminotransferase; ALT, alanine aminotransferase.

also been concern as to the long-term toxicity of regular steroids, since this paper did not discuss this issue. Therefore at this stage it makes clinical sense to await the results of further large studies before the use of low-dose corticosteroids is accepted as a routine in the management of rheumatoid arthritis.

Corticosteroids preparations

Corticosteroids are used in rheumatoid arthritis in the form of oral tablets, intra-articular and intramuscular injections and in infusion. Table 11.5 gives the equivalent doses of commonly used systemic corticosteroids.

Corticosteroid	Approximate equivalent dose
Hydrocortisone	20 mg
Prednisolone	5 mg
Deflazacort	6 mg
Methylprednisolone	4 mg
Triamcinolone	4 mg
Betamethasone	0.75 mg
Dexamethasone	0.75 mg

Table 11.5
Comparing equivalent doses of different corticosteroids

Intra-articular injections

Rheumatoid arthritis commonly involves multiple joints needing systemic treatment. However, sometimes at the initial presentation or during the flare up, one or two joints are significantly more inflamed, swollen and painful, and restrict activity. Aspiration and intra-articular corticosteroid injection of these joints can suppress synovitis for up to 3 months. The response, however, is variable and in some patients improvements last for a very short time.

A joint that is red, hot and tender should only be injected with corticosteroids after sepsis has been excluded. It is always advisable to aspirate any obvious joint effusion before injection. This alleviates discomfort caused by mechanical tension and decreases pain by decreasing the intra-articular pressure.

There are no hard and fast rules as to the frequency of injection at the same site. However, generally a single joint should not be injected more than three or four times in a year. Failure of the first injection could possibly be due to inaccurate positioning of the injection. If there is no response following the second injection, it may be that the diagnosis was incorrect or there may be a need to adjust the systemic treatment.

Generally the clinical effect of an intra-articular corticosteroid injection is of a shorter duration in joints with a large synovial cavity, such as the knee joint, because corticosteroids are more rapidly absorbed from the large synovial surface. Therefore an inflamed knee is more likely to need a repeat injection than a joint with a relatively smaller synovial cavity, such as the small joints of the hand.

If appropriate precautions are taken before and during the injection, sepsis caused by an intra-articular injection is rare, i.e. approximately 1 in 15 000 to 1 in 50 000. Since corticosteroids can facilitate bacterial growth, it is very important to use an aseptic non-touch technique.

It is always advisable to wash one's hands, preferably with an antiseptic, and then dry them thoroughly. Gloves are generally not required. Pre-packed sterilized disposable needles and syringes should be used. The skin surface could be cleaned with iodine, isopropyl alcohol or a similar antiseptic. Do not allow anything to touch the injection site once it has been cleaned and never use a finger to guide the needle into the joint. It is of prime importance not to inject a joint if there is any evidence of infection nearby.

Pulse methylprednisolone therapy

Some patients with rheumatoid arthritis with acute flare get a substantial benefit with methylprednisolone infusions. The dosing of these infusions depends on the degree of flare, but generally the dose is 200 mg to 1 g on three consecutive days.

Pulse methylprednisolone therapy is usually used in combination with a second-line agent since it has no proven disease remission properties of its own. The clinical response to methylprednisolone is usually fairly rapid and clinical improvement can last for 2–4 months.

Corticosteroids and bone

Over the past decade there has been extensive work exploring the effects of corticosteroids on bone mineral density and the use of osteoprotective agents. Low doses of corticosteroids do not appear to be a significant risk factor for the development of generalized osteoporosis; however, prolonged use of steroids does produce a decrease in bone mineral density compared to non-corticosteroid-treated patients (Sambrook *et al.*, 1986).

The reduction in bone mineral density is a major concern relating to the long-term use of corticosteroids in rheumatoid arthritis. The bone mineral loss increases after the menopause and this problem can become severe in rheumatoid arthritis patients who are also taking corticosteroids. There are published guidelines for the management of corticosteroid-induced osteoporosis (American College of Rheumatology Task Force on Osteoporosis Guidelines, 1996).

References

American College of Rheumatology Ad Hoc Committee on Guidelines (1996) Guidelines for monitoring drug therapy in rheumatoid arthritis. *Athritis Rheum.*, **39**, 723–731.

American College of Rheumatology Task Force on Osteoporosis Guidelines (1996) Recommendations for the prevention and treatment of glucorticoid-induced osteoporosis. *Arthritis Rheum.*, **39**(11), 1791–1801.

Backlund, L. and Tiselius, P. (1967) Objective measurement of joint stiffness in rheumatoid arthritis. *Acta Rheum. Scand.*, **13**, 275–288.

Banwell, B.F. (1986) Physical therapy in arthritis management, in *Rehabilitation Management of Rheumatic Conditions* (ed. G. Erlich), pp. 264–284. Williams and Wilkins, Baltimore.

Barls C.A., Lampman, R.M., Banwell, B. *et al.* (1985) Measurement of exercise tolerance in patients with rheumatoid arthritis and osteoarthritis. *J. Rheumatol.*, **12**, 458.

Carette, S., Marcoux, S. and Gingras, S. (1989) Post menopausal hormones and the incidence of rheumatoid arthritis. *J. Rheumatol.*, **16**, 911–913.

Danneskiold-Samsoe, B. and Grimby, G. (1986) Isokinetic and isometric strength in patients with rheumatoid arthritis. The relationship to clinical parameters and the influence of corticosteroids. *Clin. Rheumatol.*, **5**, 459–467.

Ekblom, B., Lovgren, O., Alderin, M. *et al.* (1974) Physical performance in patients with rheumatoid arthritis. *Scand. J. Rheumatol.*, **3**, 121–125.

Feibel, A. and Fast, A. (1976) Deep heating of joints: a consideration. *Arch. Phys. Med. Rehabil.*, **57**, 513.

Fleming, A., Crown, J.M. and Corbett, M. (1976) Early rheumatoid disease. 1. Onset. *Ann. Rheum. Dis.*, **35**, 357–360.

Garrod, A.B. (1859) *The Nature and Treatment of Gout and Rheumatoid Gout*, Walton and Maberley, London.

Hazas, J.M.W., Dijkmans, A.C., Vandendroucke, J.P. *et al.* (1990) Pregnancy and the risk of developing rheumatoid arthritis. *Arthritis Rheum.*, **33**, 1770–1775.

Kirwan, J.R. (1995) The effect of glucorticoids on joint destruction in rheumatoid arthritis. *New Engl. J. Med.*, **333**, 142–146.

Leban, M.M. (1962) Collagen tissue: implication of its response to stress in vitro. *Arch. Phys. Med. Rehabil.*, **43**, 461–466.

Linos, A., Worthington, J.W., O'Fallon, W.M. *et al.* (1980) The epidemiology of rheumatoid arthritis in Rochester, Minnosota: a study of incidence, prevalence and mortality. *Am. J. Epedemiol.*, **111**, 87–98.

McConkey, B., Crockson, R.A., Crockson, A.P. *et al.* (1973) The effect of some anti-inflammatory drugs on the acute phase proteins in rheumatoid arthritis. *Quart. J. Med.*, **42**, 785–792.

Myllykangas-Luosujarvi, R.A., Aho, K. and Isomaki, H.A. (1995a) Data attributed to antirheumatic medication in a nation wide series of 1,666 patients with rheumatoid .arthritis who have died. *J. Rheumatol.*, **22**, 2214–2217.

Myllykangas-Luosujarvi, R.A., Aho, K., Isomaki, H.A. (1995b) Mortality in rheumatoid arthritis. *Semin. Arthritis Rheum.*, **25**, 193–202.

Nepom, J.T., Hansen, J.A. and Nepom, B.S. (1987) The molecular basis for HLA class 2 associations with rheumatoid arthritis. *J. Clin. Immunol.*, **7**, 1–7.

Nicholas, M.S. and Panayi, G.S. (1988) Rheumatoid arthritis and pregnancy. *Clin. Exp. Rheumatol.*, **6**, 179–182.

Nordesjo, L.O., Nordgren, V. and Wigren, A. (1983) Isometric strength and endurance in patients with severe rheumatoid arthritis or osteoarthritis in the knee joint. *Scand. J. Rheumatol.*, **12**, 152–156.

Sambrook, P.N., Eisman, J.A., Yeates, M.G. *et al.* (1986) Osteoporosis in rheumatoid arthritis; safety of low dose corticosteroids. *Ann. Rheum. Dis.*, **45**, 950–953.

Smith, C.A. and Arnett, S. (1991) Epidemiologic aspects of rheumatoid arthritis: Current immunogenetic approach. *Clin. Orthop.*, **265**, 23–35.

Snorrason, E. (1952) Landre-Beauvais and his goutte asthenique primitive. *Acta Med. Scand.*, **142**, Suppl. 266, 115–118.

Spector, T., Brennen, P., Harris, B. *et al.* (1991) Does oestrogen replacement therapy protect against rheumatoid arthritis? *J. Rheumatol.*, **18**, 1473–1476.

Symmond, D. (1995) Excess mortality in rheumatoid arthritis: Is it the disease or the drugs ? *J. Rheumatol.*, **22**, 2200–2202.

Symmons, D.P.M. (1998) Mortality in rheumatoid arthritis. *Br. J. Rheumatol.*, **27**, Suppl., 44–54.

Warren, C.G., Lehmann, J.F. and Koblanski, J.N. (1976) Heat and stretch procedures: an evaluation using rat tail tendons. *Arch. Phys. Med. Rehabil.*, **57**, 122–126.

Wicks, I.P., Moore, J. and Fleming, A. (1988) Australian mortality statistics for rheumatoid arthritis 1950–1981: analysis of death certificate data. *Ann. Rheum. Dis.*, **47**, 569.

Osteoarthritis

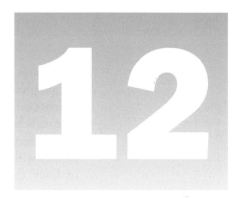

Osteoarthritis, which means inflammation of bone and joint, is sometimes also called 'degenerative joint disease' or 'osteoarthrosis'. The later two terminologies consider osteoarthritis to be a 'wear and tear' or non-inflammatory arthropathy. The term osteoarthritis, however, is most widely used.

The prevalence of osteoarthritis increases with age. In the Western world about 80% of people above the age of 75 years have radiological evidence of osteoarthritis. Osteoarthritis is more common among women. Age-related osteoarthritis is usually generalized, with some joints more painful than the others. Premature osteoarthritis in a single joint usually follows localized severe or repetitive trauma. The other individual risk factors for osteoarthritis include obesity, hypermobile joints and certain occupations; knee osteoarthritis, for example, occurs more frequently in coal miners (Kellergen and Lawrence, 1952), dockers (Partridge and Duthie, 1968) and shipyard workers (Lindberg and Montgomery, 1987). There is also a possible association of localized osteoarthritis in certain sports such as football, rugby and weight lifting (Panush and Brown, 1987). Some clinicians prefer to divide the disorder into primary or idiopathic and secondary osteoarthritis.

Pathophysiology

The pathophysiology of osteoarthritis is loosely defined and a strong emphasis is still placed on age-related degenerative changes of cartilage as the cardinal feature of this disorder. The suffix 'itis' implies inflammation at the cellular level. Changes in osteoarthritis usually involve all the tissues that form the synovial joint, including articular cartilage, subchondral bone and synovium, and adjoining soft tissues, including ligaments, joint capsule and muscles acting on the particular joint.

The initial visible radiological sign of osteoarthritis is loss of cartilage. This occurs in the form of localized disruption of the most superficial layers of the articular cartilage, with localized fibrillation and degradation. With the progression of the disease, the articular surface becomes irregular and changes extend deeper into the cartilage, resulting in deep fissures and tears. The subchondral bone changes usually accompany the changes in the deeper part of articular cartilage and include increased subchondral bone density with remodelling of subchondral bone. This results in the formation of bony cysts of variable size and subchondral sclerosis. As the disease progresses, the articular cartilage is almost completely lost, resulting in one bone rubbing against the opposite denuded bony surface.

The osteophytes and soft tissue growth at the joint margins usually accompany the changes in the articular cartilage and subchondral bone. The commonest site for these osteophytes is around the periphery of the joint at the cartilage–bone interface, but they can also form along the joint capsule insertion. The exact mechanism responsible for osteophyte formation remains unknown, but it is presumably the result of remodelling in response to degenerative changes in the articular cartilage and subchondral bone.

The changes in the cartilage and subchondral bone distort the normal shape of the joint, which results in secondary changes in the synovium or joint capsule and the ligaments and muscles around the involved joint. Inflammation of the synovium can result in joint effusion. With the passage of time the joint capsule and ligaments become contracted. The pain in the joint results in a decreased range of motion, which leads to secondary muscle atrophy resulting in joint instability, stiffness and weakness.

Possible causes of pain in osteoarthritis

Pain with tenderness and stiffness of variable degree is the most commonly reported symptom in osteoarthritis. The normal joint function is impaired. The freedom of movement of smooth articular surfaces is removed by an irregular rough cartilage surface with a decreased joint space. This leads to an imbalance of the load distribution across the joint tissue, resulting in instability of the joint.

Most joints have a good nerve supply to the synovium and the joint capsule. The nerve fibres act as pain receptors and mechanoreceptors and have a role in the protective reflexes that prevent potentially damaging joint movement. The peripheral part of the menisci also has a nerve supply and the subchondral bone has perivascular nerves.

Several possible pathological mechanisms for pain in osteoarthritis have been suggested, including inflammatory synovitis, increased intraosseous pressure, periosteal elevation and changes in the periarticular structures, including capsules, ligaments and muscles. It has been suggested that increased intraosseous pressure is responsible for severe prolonged pain at night and during rest.

The exact mechanism of raised intraosseous pressure is unknown, but it could be secondary to obstruction of venous outflow (Arnoldi, Lempberg and Linderholm, 1971; Arnoldi *et al.*, 1980). Mild inflammation of the synovium commonly occurs in osteoarthritis and is one of the contributing factors to pain and stiffness. Changes in the soft structures around the joint can lead to tenosynovitis and bursitis. Moderately severe osteoarthritis can also lead to muscle and ligament weakness. Exercises to strengthen the muscles around the joint stabilize the relevant joint and also decrease the mechanical pain of osteoarthritis (Chamberlain, Care and Harfield, 1982; Puett and Griffin, 1992). In addition to local factors, spinal and central mechanisms may augment the pain in patients with osteoarthritis. There is also an association between osteoarthritis and fibromyalgia (Moldofsky, 1989) and depression and anxiety (Summers *et al.*, 1988).

Clinical features

Pain with stiffness and tenderness are cardinal features of osteoarthritis. The osteoarthritic pain is usually associated with the presence of radiological changes. There is also an association with low socioeconomic status (Hochberg *et al.*, 1989; Davis *et al.*, 1991; Bradley, 1994). A study comparing knee pain among the poor and the affluent found a significantly higher frequency of pain in the latter, which increased with age and was more common in females. This study also noted that squatting was more common in the poor, but did not find any relation between knee pain and joint laxity (Gibson *et al.*, 1996).

There appears to be a poor correlation between radiographic evidence of osteoarthritis and pain. Osteoarthritis in the small joints of the hands is least likely to give pain (excluding the base of the thumb), while the correlation between pain and osteoarthritis of the hip is more significant. The severity of pain in osteoarthritis increases with advanced radiographic changes, though occasionally severe joint damage can be asymptomatic (Hochberg *et al.*, 1989). The pain in the majority of cases is use related, but about 30–50% of patients get pain even at rest and at night (Cushnaghan, 1991).

Examination findings usually depend on the severity of the osteoarthritis. There may be an obvious bony swelling with or without an effusion. Mild tenderness over the joint line is very common, as is crepitus. The range of movements at a particular joint may be limited and painful. There may be features of periarticular involvement contributing to pain such as tenosynovitis, bursitis or pain at the insertion of ligaments supporting the joint.

Advanced osteoarthritis usually leads to instability of the weight-bearing joint.

Management

Osteoarthritis is a heterogeneous group of conditions which is extremely common. The commonest sites of involvement are knees, hips, hands and the facet joints of the spine. At present there is no specific treatment available that significantly alters the natural course of the disease. There are certain key questions for future research, such as the effect of pain control on the natural progression of osteoarthritis.

Pain in osteoarthritis is frequently under-assessed and inadequately treated. A good history followed by complete examination should be a prerequisite for treatment. There is usually a lack of communication between patient and treating doctor regarding their personal views on the importance of pain and its alleviation (Dieppe and Cushnaghan, 1992). From the patient's perspective the most important aspect is often the relief of pain. Osteoarthritis is incurable and it is therefore important that the treatment aims to reduce the pain, thereby increasing mobility, and to limit further joint damage. Table 12.1 summarizes the management of osteoarthritis. This can be divided into three categories: non-pharmacological, pharmacological and surgical.

Table 12.1
Management of painful osteoarthritis

Non-pharmacological
- Patient education
- Physiotherapy
- Occupational therapy
- Self-help groups

Pharmacological
Simple analgesics
- Non-opioids
- Non-steroidal anti-inflammatory drugs
- Topical analgesics

Opioid analgesics
Short course of antidepressants
Intra-articular corticosteroid injections

Surgery

NON-PHARMACOLOGICAL INTERVENTIONS

Patient education

Patient education is the most important part of the management of osteoarthritis. For a successful outcome it is very important for patients to be aware of the diagnosis, prognosis and factors with major impact on outcome. Patients should be encouraged to lose weight and if appropriate be referred for dietetic advice and regular monitoring. Weight loss is associated with an improvement in the symptoms of knee osteoarthritis (Loseser *et al.*, 1995), though it is not known whether it has any significant effect on the progression of the existing disease.

Many patients are concerned as to the detrimental effect of exercise on their joints. Patients should be encouraged to exercise where possible to increase the muscle strength and range of movement around the affected joint. The exercise programme, however, should be appropriate for each patient. Knee pain due to patellofemoral osteoarthritis may get worse with cycling, and taping the patella in a medial position may give a short-term relief in patients with this condition (Cushnaghan, McCarthy and Dieppe, 1994). Similarly swimming may ease back and hip pain but can aggravate neck pain due to cervical facet osteoarthritis.

Patient education could be in the form of simple explanation with backup advice from an information leaflet. Self-management programmes with the help of a practice or district nurse and help-line telephone number improve patients' long-term health and reduce the frequency of medical consultations.

Role of physiotherapist

The management of osteoarthritis is a team effort in which physiotherapy and occupational therapy play a major part, particularly in those patients with moderate to severe osteoarthritis of large joints.

Physiotherapists play an important part in maintaining the range of motion of a joint with exercises to increase muscle strength acting on a particular joint. Increasing range of motion and muscle strength stabilizes the joint, which decreases pain and increases mobility. Hydrotherapy can play an important part in pain relief and muscle relaxation. A quadriceps muscle strengthening exercise programme can diminish pain and increase mobility in patients with knee osteoarthritis (Puett and Griffin, 1994).

Role of occupational therapist

Occupational therapy goes hand in hand with physiotherapy. Occupational therapists play an important part in teaching joint protection technique and coping strategies. People with osteoarthritic joints are provided with a variety of aids, including walking sticks, arthroses and splints. Some patients are a poor risk for surgery and in these patients with advanced osteoarthritis splints may help in stability and mobility (Hicks and Gerber, 1992). Sometimes simple shoe modification can decrease pain and increase the mobility by reducing impact loading on lower limb joints.

PHARMACOLOGICAL TREATMENT

The choice of an analgesic depends on many factors, including the severity of pain, efficacy, tolerance and the safety profile of the drug. Drug therapy for osteoarthritis is largely administered orally; other routes include rectal, topical, intra-articular and intramuscular (Table 12.2).

There are various drugs belonging to different chemical groups currently used in the management of osteoarthritis with variable results. The majority of these agents are non-specific and largely used for pain relief. However, some agents have recently been used with a 'chondro-protective effect'.

The majority of patients with mild osteoarthritis get good relief from a simple analgesic such as paracetamol, a low-dose salicylate, codeine or a combination of these agents, or from a non-steroidal anti-inflammatory

Table 12.2

Routes of administration of analgesics for osteoarthritis

Oral
- Tablets (paracetamol)
- Capsules (etodolac)
- Suspensions (paracetamol)
- Sublingual (buprenorphine)

Rectal
- Suppository (paracetamol, diclofenac sodium, morphine)

Topical
- Non-steroidal anti-inflammatory drugs (gels and creams)
- Capsaicin
- Methyl salicylate

Intra-articular
- Corticosteroids (triamcinolone)
- Chondroprotective agents (hyaluronan)

Intramuscular (for acute pain)

Intravenous (for chronic pain)
- Lidocaine infusion

drug (NSAID). Stronger opioids should not be used routinely, though a short course of dihydrocodeine or codeine in a single or compound preparation with paracetamol may be helpful to control acute pain. Table 12.3 lists the analgesics commonly used in the management of osteoarthritis.

NSAIDs are the most commonly used drugs for the treatment of osteoarthritis. There is substantial evidence to show their superiority over placebo in osteoarthritis (Dieppe *et al.*, 1993). However, there are very few comparative studies of NSAIDs and simple analgesics (Brooks, Potter and Buchanan, 1982; Bradley *et al.*, 1991). Mild to moderate osteoarthritis patients get a good response with paracetamol only (Dieppe *et al.*, 1993; Williams *et al.*, 1993). A recent study did not find any significant difference between paracetamol and ibuprofen in symptom relief (Bradley, 1994).

The use of pharmacological agents in the management of osteoarthritis is not clear (McAlindon and Dieppe, 1990; Liang and Fortin, 1991) and there has been concern over the adverse effects of NSAIDs on articular cartilage (Doherty and Dieppe, 1981; Ghosh, 1989). The rationale for using NSAIDs for the treatment of osteoarthritis is to treat the inflammatory component. Practically, however, it is very difficult to assess whether an osteoarthritic joint has any significant inflammation. However, patients without synovitis may also benefit from taking NSAIDs (Brandt, 1993). Since the pain of osteoarthritis may remit and relapse, it is important to

Drug category	Example
Simple analgesics	Paracetamol and aspirin. Patients with mild pain usually respond to these analgesics
Non-steroidal anti-inflammatory drugs	Ibuprofen, diclofenac sodium, etc. NSAIDs are often required when there is inflammation. Potentially series side-effects. Give short courses.
Opioids	Codeine and dihydrocodeine. For moderate to severe pain associated with osteoarthritis. Their use is limited because of side-effects such as nausea, vomiting, constipation, drowsiness and addiction. Give short courses.
Intra-articular corticosteroids	Triamcinolone. Useful when there is associated synovitis. These drugs should be used sparingly.

Table 12.3
Commonly used analgesics for the treatment of osteoarthritis

regularly review medications and titrate according to the severity of the symptoms.

NSAIDs are potentially toxic, with well-known serious gastrointestinal, renal and hepatic side-effects. Osteoarthritis is most common in the elderly population, who are also at risk of serious gastrointestinal and other side-effects from these drugs. The gastric side-effect profile is variable and in some NSAIDs, such as nabumetone, meloxicam and etodolac, they are thought to be less severe. Gastric protection in susceptible patients can be provided by an H_2 antagonist, proton pump inhibitor or prostaglandin analogue, such as misoprostol. The gastric protection provided by all these agents is incomplete and therefore NSAIDs should still be used with caution in the elderly population.

The simple analgesics can be used on an 'as required' basis or can be taken on a regular basis with good effect, but for NSAIDs regular prescribing rather than on an 'as required' usage is recommended. It is, however, prudent to use courses of NSAIDs for a few weeks only with simple analgesics to avoid serious side-effects.

NSAIDs are also available in the form of gels and creams, intramuscular injections and suppositories. The local applicants, such as gels and creams, have been shown in trials to give symptomatic relief for monoarticular disease and those diseases with involvement of the small joints of the hands (Norris and Guttadauna, 1987). NSAID gels and creams are relatively expensive and so far their clinical efficacy in generalized osteoarthritis remains unproved.

Corticosteroids

There is no place for systemic corticosteroids in the management of osteoarthritis. However, patients with osteoarthritis at the base of thumb and those with an inflammatory component, such as a small effusion, may get a good response to an intra-articular corticosteroid. It is very important to aspirate an effusion in a joint prior to the injection to get maximum benefit. Also physiotherapy on its own is unlikely to be fully successful in the presence of an effusion as it can result in loss of muscle strength (Faher *et al.*, 1988). There is evidence that the clinical response to an intra-articular injection is enhanced if the injected joint is rested for 1 or 2 days following the injection.

Other drugs

Large numbers of other agents have been used for the management of osteoarthritis. A small controlled study of intra-articular yttrium-90 injections into the knee associated with chondrocalcinosis reported more symptomatic improvement in the injected joint than in the controlled knee over a 6 month period (Doherty and Dieppe, 1981). There is also some anecdotal evidence of uncontrolled observation suggesting a longer-lasting benefit of yttrium injections for simple osteoarthritis of the knee. This treatment, however, is not at this stage recommended for general use and there is a need for more well-controlled long-term studies.

In some countries some chondro-protective agents have been used with long-term benefits in human hip and knee osteoarthritis (Ragholec, 1987). The agents most commonly used include glycosaminoglycan polysulphate ester, glycosaminoglycan-peptide complex and hyaluronan. These agents have essentially important in vitro effects on animal models. So far there is a paucity of data on controlled trials in human osteoarthritis.

There is a limited role for other agents, such as appetite suppressants and antidepressants in the management of osteoarthritis. Some studies have reported benefit from intra-articular injections of morphine (Likar *et al.*, 1997). There has also been a report on pain relief with intra-articular injections of superoxide dismutase inhibitor orgotein (Mazierres, Maskoue-lier and Capron, 1991).

Topical capsaicin cream has been reported to be better than placebo in providing pain relief in osteoarthritis (Deal *et al.*, 1991; Altman *et al.*, 1994; Zhange and Li Wan, 1994). There is some evidence that a higher strength capsaicin may work more quickly than the milder form in relieving the pain of osteoarthritis (Schnitzer, Posner and Lawrence, 1995). Capsaicin produces analgesia by depleting sensory neurones of the pain neurotransmitter substance P.

SURGERY

Some patients with osteoarthritic knee pain may benefit from a non-arthroscopic washout, i.e. closed tidal irrigation (Ike *et al.*, 1992), or arthroscopic washout and cartilage debridement.

Patients with severe osteoarthritis, persistent pain and associated disability not responding to conservative management usually require surgery. The joints most commonly requiring surgery are the knee and hip. The outcome following knee and hip replacement is good, particularly in those with no preoperative medical illness and perioperative and postoperative complications.

References

Altman, R.D., Aven, A., Holmburg, C.E. *et al.* (1994) Capsaicin cream 0.025% as monotherapy for osteoarthritis: a double blind study. *Semin. Arthritis Rheum.*, **23**, Suppl 3, 25–33.

Arnoldi, C.C., Djurhws, J.C., Heelfordt, J. *et al.* (1980) Interosseous phlebography, interosseous pressure measurement and Tc (m) – polyphosphate scintigraphy in patients with various painful conditions in the hip and knee. *Acta Orthop. Scand.*, **51**, 19–28.

Arnoldi, C.C., Lempberg, R.K. and Linderholm, H. (1971) Immediate effect of osteotomy on the intra-medullary pressure of the femoral head and neck in patients with degenerative osteoarthritis. *Acta Orthop. Scand.*, **42**, 357–365.

Bradley, J.D., Brandt, K.D., Katz, B.P. *et al.* (1991) Comparison of an anti-inflammatory dose of ibuprofen and analgesic dose of ibuprofen and acetaminophen in the treatment of patients with osteoarthritis of the knee. *N. Engl. J. Med.*, **325**, 87–91.

Bradley, L.A. (1994) Psychological dimensions of rheumatoid arthritis, in *Rheumatoid Arthritis: Pathogenesis, Assessment, Outcome and Treatment.* (eds F. Wolfe and T. Bincus), Marcel Dekker, New York.

Brandt, K.D. (1993) Should osteoarthritis be treated with nonsteroidal antiinflammatory drugs? *Rheum. Dis. Clin. N. Am.*, **19**, 697–712.

Brooks, P.M., Potter, S.R. and Buchanan, W.W. (1982) NSAIDs and osteoarthritis – help or hindrance? *J. Rheumatol.*, **9**, 3–5.

Chamberlain, M.A., Care, G. and Harfield, B. (1982) Physiotherapy in osteoarthritis of knee: a control trial of hospital versus home exercises. *Int. Rehabil. Med.*, **4**, 191–206.

Cushnaghan, J. (1991) Osteoarthritis: a clinical and radiological study. MSc thesis, Bristol University.

Cushnaghan, J., McCarthy, C. and Dieppe, P. (1994) Taping the patella medially: a new treatment for osteoarthritis of the knee. *Br. Med. J.*, **308**, 753–755.

Davis, M.A., Ettinger, W.H., Newhaus, J.M. *et al.* (1991) Knee osteoarthritis and physical functioning: evidence from the NHANES I epidemiologic follow up study. *J. Rheumatol.*, **18**, 591–598.

Deal, C.L., Schnitzer, T.J., Lipstein, E. *et al.* (1991) Treatment of arthritis with topical capsaicin: a double blind trial. *Clin. Ther.*, **13**, 383–395.

Dieppe, P. and Cushnaghan, J. (1992) The natural course and prognosis of osteoarthritis, in *Osteoarthritis*, 2nd edn (eds R. Moskowitz, D. Howell, V. Goldberg and H. Mankin), pp. 399–412. W.B Saunders, Philadelphia.

Dieppe, P., Cushnaghan, J., Jasani, M.K. *et al.* (1993) A two year placebo controlled trial of non-steroidal anti-inflammatory therapy in osteoarthritis of the knee. *Brit. J. Rheumatol.*, **35**, 595–600.

Doherty, M. and Dieppe, P. (1981) Effect of intra-articular yttrium 90 on chronic pyrophosphate arthropathy (CPA) of the knee. *Lancet*, 1243–1245.

Faher, H., Rentsch, H.W., Gerber, N.J. *et al.* (1988) Knee effusion and reflex inhibition of quadriceps. *J. Bone Joint Surg.*, **70B**, 635–637.

Ghosh, P. (1989) Anti rheumatic drugs and cartilage. *Baillière's Clin. Rheumatol.*, **2**, 309–338.

Gibson, T., Hameed, K., Kadir, M. *et al.* (1996) Knee pain amongst the poor and affluent in Pakistan. *Br. J. Rheumatol.*, **35**(2), 146–149.

Hicks, J.E. and Gerber, L.X. (1992) Rehabilitation in the management of patients with osteoarthritis, *Osteoarthritis*, 2nd edn (eds R. Moskowitz, D. Howell, V. Goldberg and H. Mankin), pp. 427–464. W.B. Saunders, Philadelphia.

Hochberg, M.C., Lawrence, R.C., Evrett, D.F. *et al.* (1989) Epidemiologic associations of pain in osteoarthritis of the knee. Data from the National Health and Nutrition survey and the National Health and Nutrition examination. Epidemiologic follow up survey. *Semin. Arthritis Rheum.*, **18** (4, Suppl. p. 2), 4–9.

Ike, R.W., Arnold, W.J., Rothschild, E.W. *et al.* (1992) The tidal irrigation co-operating group. Tidal irrigation versus conservative medical management in patients with osteoarthritis of the knee: a prospective randomised study. *J. Rheumatol.*, **19**, 772–779.

Kellergen, J.H. and Lawrence, J.S. (1952) Rheumatism in miners. Part II: X-ray study. *Br. J. Ind. Med.*, **9**, 197–207.

Liang, M.H. and Fortin, P. (1991) Management of osteoarthritis of the hip and knee. *N. Engl. J. Med.*, **325**, 125–127.

Likar, R., Schafer, M., Paulak, F. *et al.* (1997) Intra-articular morphine analgesia in chronic pain patients with osteoarthritis. *Anaesthesia and Analgesia*, **84**(6), 1313–1317.

Lindberg, H. and Montgomery, F. (1987) Heavy labour and occurrence of gonarthosis. *Clin. Orthop.*, **214**, 235–236.

Loseser, K., Niklas B.J., Bunyard, L.B. *et al.* (1995) The effect of an exercise and weight loss intervention on osteoarthritis of knee. *Arthritis Rheum.*, **38**, Suppl. 9,/S268 (abstract).

Mazieres, B., Maskouelier, A.M. and Capron, M.H. (1991) A French controlled multi-centre study of intra-articular orgotein versus intra-articular corticosteroids in the treatment of knee osteoarthritis: a one year follow-up. *J. Rheumatol.*, **18**, 134–137.

McAlindon, T. and Dieppe, P. (1990) The medical management of osteoarthritis of the knee: an inflammatory issue? *Br. J. Rheumatol.*, **29**, 471–473.

Moldofsky, H. (1989) Sleep influences on regional and diffuse pain syndromes associated with osteoarthritis. *Semin. Arthritis Rheum.*, **18**, Suppl. 2, 18–21.

Norris, E. and Guttadauna, M. (1987) Piroxicam: new dosage form. *Eur. J. Rheumatol. Inflamm.*, **8**, 94–104.

Panush, R.S. and Brown, D.G. (1987) Exercise and arthritis. *Sports Med.*, **4**, 54–64.

Partridge, R.E.H. and Duthie, J.J.R. (1968) Rheumatism in dockers and civil servants: a comparison of heavy manual and sedentary workers. *Ann. Rheum. Dis.*, **27**, 559–568.

Puett, D.W. and Griffin, M.R. (1992) Published trials of nonmedicinal and non-invasive therapies for hip and knee osteoarthritis. *Ann. Intern. Med.*, **116**, 529–534.

Puett, D.W. and Griffin, M.R. (1994) Published trials of nonmedicinal and non-invasive therapies for hip and knee osteoarthritis *Ann. Intern. Med.*, **121**, 133–140.

Ragholec, W. (1987) Long-term studies of anti-osteoarthritic drugs: an assessment. *Semin. Arthritis Rheum.*, **17**, Suppl. 1, 3–34.

Schnitzer, T.J., Posner, M. and Lawrence, I.D. (1995) High strength capsaicin cream for osteoarthritis pain: rapid onset of the action and improved efficacy with twice daily dosing. *J. Clin. Rheumatol.*, **1**, 268–273.

Summers, M.N., Haley, W.E., Reveille, J.O. *et al.* (1988) Radiographic assessment and psychological variables as predictors of pain and functional impairment in osteoarthritis of the knee or hip. *Arthritis Rheum.*, **31**, 204–209.

Williams, H.J., Ward, J.R., Egger, M.J. *et al.* (1993) Comparison of naproxen and acetaminophen in a two year study of treatment of osteoarthritis of knee. *Arthritis Rheum.*, **36**, 1196–2006.

Zhange, W.Y. and Li Wan P.O.A. (1994) The effectiveness of topically applied capsaicin. A meta analysis. *Eur. J. Clin. Pharmacol.*, **46**(6), 517–522.

Low back pain

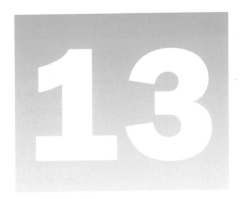

Low back pain is very common and most of us suffer self-limiting back pain sometime during our lives. There is no universally accepted anatomical definition of low back pain but it can be defined as 'pain arising from the posterior region of the trunk within an area bounded more or less by sagittal planes tangential to the lateral borders of the erector spinae, a transverse plane through the T12 spinous processes and a transverse plane through the posterior superior iliac spines' (Bogduk, 1992).

The spine is divided into four anatomical regions, i.e. 7 cervical vertebrae, 12 thoracic vertebrae, 5 lumbar vertebrae, and 5 fused sacral vertebrae and a coccygeal segment. The lumbar spine connects the thoracic spine with the pelvis and is responsible for movements, including flexion, extension, rotation and lateral bending. The lower segment of the lumbar spine absorbs high loading pressure, is involved in rotational movement and is the commonest site of low back pain.

The intervertebral disc has two components: a soft nucleus pulposus and a surrounding by annulus fibrosus. The disc acts as a cushion between the adjacent vertebra and has a scant nerve supply to its peripheral parts. Increased intradiscal pressure also leads to back pain, suggesting the presence of pressure receptors in the central part of the disc. Adjacent vertebrae articulate with two facet joints on each side of the vertebral body. The facet joint is a synovial joint and has its own nerve supply, and is commonly a source of pain.

Epidemiology

Most episodes of back pain are of short duration and about 75% of patients with acute low back pain improve in 4 weeks (Spitzer et al., 1987). The annual incidence of back pain is about 5% and its prevalence is 60–80% (Damkot et al., 1984; Frymoyar and Cats-Baril, 1991). The frequency of back pain reported is different between different communities (Papageorgiou et al., 1995; Carey et al., 1996).

The terminology commonly used to describe low back pain includes acute low back pain, i.e. pain of 0–7 days' duration, while back pain of more than 3 months' duration is defined as chronic back pain. The other terminologies include intractable pain and low back pain with sciatica.

There are a number of risk factors associated with low back pain. Although osteoarthritis and radiological changes in the spine increase with age, the proportion of patients reporting low back pain is highest in early adult life and in the forties and fifties. The reason for a decline in reporting of this condition in the elderly is not known. Low back pain of mechanical origin is uncommon in children. Low back pain is reported more by women than men, and sciatica is commoner in men. Low back pain is more common in smokers. The other individual risk factor include history of pregnancy, trauma, employment in a heavy manual jobs involving lifting and carrying of heavy weights along with twisting movements of the spine, and also anxiety and depression.

Sources of low back pain

The main sources of back pain are the intervertebral disc, facet joints and spinal nerve root. Neurogenic low back pain can arise from pressure on the intravertebral nerve root at various sites, such as a disc herniation, pressure on the nerve root from the osteophytes or hypertrophy of the facet joint. Table 13.1 lists the sources of low back pain.

Clinical evaluation

The intensity of back pain varies greatly. In some patients it leads to debilitating symptoms affecting their social and personal life, while in others it is a nagging discomfort that is made worse by certain activities. There are many sources of low back pain with some characteristic features. To identify the possible source of pain a detailed medical history and physical examination remains the main tool. A large proportion of patients with low back pain do not need any further evaluation with plain X-rays or expensive imaging.

The important points in the history of low back pain include duration (acute or chronic or acute on chronic), nature (dull, sharp, etc.), radiation, aggravating and relieving factors, fever, weight loss, and effect on daily life including hobbies and work (Table 13.2).

The back pain of disc or facet joint origin is usually localized in the lumbar area, but can radiate into the buttocks and down to the mid-thigh. The character of this pain varies from a deep-rooted dull ache to a sharp pain. The pain from the facet joint is usually made worse on extension and rotational movement of the lumbar spine and can be localized by deep pressure over the corresponding facet joint. Back pain of any origin can lead to paravertebral muscle spasm with stiffening, and abnormal posture, including diminished lumbar lordosis.

Radicular pain usually radiates into one leg and most commonly affects the L4/5 lumbar nerve root. The intensity of the pain is quite severe and usually radiates along the corresponding dermatome. Radicular pain may be associated with paresthesias and weakness in the corresponding leg. These

Table 13.1
Sources of low back pain

Source of pain	Description
Skin and subcutaneous tissue	Trigger spots
Paraspinal muscles, fascia and ligaments	These structures are well innervated and usually produce a dull ache which is deep rooted
Facet and sacroiliac joints	Facet and sacroiliac joints are well innervated. Facet joints are a common source of mechanical low back pain. Sacroiliac joint involvement is common in seronegative spondarthropathies
Bones	Vertebral osteoporotic crush fractures; osteomalacia; Paget's disease
Disc	Deep-rooted pain associated with disc herniation; discitis
Radicular	Usually sharp, shooting pain, which radiates along the dermatome of the corresponding nerve
Referred	Visceral referred pain, which lies in a viscus such as the pancreas, aorta or pelvic viscera; it is referred to as a boring, colicky or tearing pain
Neoplastic	Multiple myeloma; secondary and primary bone tumours. The quality and intensity of the pain varies from a dull deep-rooted pain to a sharp pain of vertebral collapse or a neurogenic pain.
Psychogenic	Variable character

Table 13.2
Diagnostic triage for low
back pain

Medical history

Site
> Localized to a particular point such as facet joint or diffuse

Duration
> Acute, chronic, acute on chronic or intractable

Nature
> Dull localized, sharp and shooting or burning

Radiation
> Radicular or localized

Aggravating factors
> Posture, valsalva manoeuvre

Relieving factors
> Rest, specific posture, local application of heat or cold

Medication
> Analgesics, etc.

Systemic complaints
> Fever, loss of appetite, weight loss, previous history of
> malignancy

symptoms are usually made worse on coughing, sneezing and laughing. The lumbar spinal movements are diminished, with restriction of straight leg raising, and symptoms are made worse on sciatic or femoral stretch testing. Ankle or knee reflexes may be diminished or absent, suggesting significant nerve root compression.

Back pain can be referred from abdominal structures and it is also important to exclude malignancy or infection in patients with severe persistent back pain associated with loss of appetite, weight loss and night sweats. Table 13.3 lists the possible causes of serious spinal pathology.

Management of low back pain

Most patients with acute low back pain improve within a few weeks and may not seek medical advice. The important steps in those requiring medical consultation are:

- patient education
- non-pharmacological therapy

Age	Severe low back pain in those under the age of 20 or above the age of 55 years
Recent trauma	Road traffic accident Fall from height Contact sport, e.g. rugby
Site	Severe thoracic or upper lumbar pain
Systemic	Anorexia, weight loss Fever, night sweats, rigors Sphincter abnormalities, i.e. difficulty in micturition Saddle anaethesia Muscle weakness and gait abnormalities Spinal structural deformity
Medications	Systemic use of corticosteroids (may cause vertebral osteoporotic fracture) Drug abuse, HIV
Past medical history	Carcinoma

Table 13.3
Possible causes of serious spinal pathology

- pharmacological therapy
- surgery.

PATIENT EDUCATION

Although most episodes of low back pain settle spontaneously, those suffering from the condition for the first time are unlikely to be aware of the long-term prognosis. They are also unlikely to have an insight as to the likely cause of their symptoms and may be frightened as to the possibility of a sinister cause or fear losing their job and long-term disability.

After a detailed history and examination the possible cause of the back pain should be explained. A small minority of patients may need further investigations to clarify the diagnosis and this should be explained in simple layman's language. Technical terms such as 'degenerative' or 'facet' joint pain should be avoided. A model of the back is usually very helpful in explaining simple anatomy and the likely sources of pain.

The doctor–patient relationship plays an important role in the patient's recovery. The role played by the family in these circumstances is not clear but those presenting with severe back pain and those with chronic back pain may benefit from a multidisciplinary approach including family support. Patients with chronic debilitating low back pain very commonly have psychosocial factors contributing to their symptoms and in these cases family support is usually very helpful.

NON-PHARMACOLOGICAL THERAPY

Physical modalities

Physiotherapy is a very important aspect of the management of low back pain. Physiotherapists should be involved early on during the course of the condition to correct the posture and to gradually mobilize the spine. In a selected group of patients with low back pain gentle spinal manipulation may be very helpful (Assendelft *et al.*, 1995).

The physiotherapy exercises should be tailor-made for each patient and include flexion and extension of the lumbar spine, stretching and aerobic conditioning. The other forms of treatment include diathermy, ultrasound, acupuncture, lumbosacral support, hot and cold packs, and transcutaneous electric nerve stimulation (TNS). The role of TNS, however, is not well established and it should not be used routinely for patients with lower back pain.

PHARMACOLOGICAL THERAPY

Drug therapy for back pain

Simple back pain is usually treated by the patient taking analgesics that are available over the counter. The majority of patients with low back pain do not need more than a few weeks' use of simple analgesia. The agents most commonly used include:

- simple analgesics
- NSAIDs
- opioid analgesics.

Paracetamol or aspirin is the 'drug of choice for simple low back pain of mild severity. Patients with moderate to severe back pain usually require additional analgesics, as paracetamol or aspirin is unlikely to achieve adequate pain control on its own. Adequate pain relief should be the initial aim of treatment, as patients are unlikely to co-operate with mobilizing exercises if in pain. Most patients with back pain do not need bed rest and should be encouraged to mobilize. A small minority with very severe low back pain and those with root symptoms may need bed rest for a short period, i.e. 2–3 days.

Non-steroidal anti-inflammatory drugs (NSAIDs) are very effective for pain relief of mild to moderate severity, particularly in patients with marked stiffness. For mild pain NSAIDs are better in combination with para-cetamol, and for those patients with moderate to severe pain they are better in combination with an opioid, such as dihydrocodeine. NSAIDs should be used with caution, particularly in the elderly and in those patients with a significant present or past history of dyspepsia, and they should be used for a short interval only.

For moderate pain not responding to paracetamol, aspirin or an NSAID, the choice of analgesics is fairly wide. Nefopam 30 mg three times a day may be helpful. Nefopam, unlike the other centrally acting analgesics, does not cause serious respiratory depression and has very minimal addiction potential.

Both paracetamol and aspirin are available in compound analgesic preparations. Co-codamol, Tylex and Co-dydramol are frequently used, particularly in patients with chronic low back pain.

If possible, it is better to avoid using opioid analgesics such as morphine and diamorphine for patients with back pain. However, other opioid analgesics such as dihydrocodeine and meptazinol are quite frequently used. The usual dose of dihydrocodeine is 30 mg every 4–6 hours. Meptazinol is also short acting, with a duration of action of 2–7 hours. Chronic opioid analgesic therapy should, if possible, be avoided and the use of opioids should be limited to patients with chronic persistent low back pain who are unlikely to benefit from surgery.

Tramadol is a strong analgesic and claims to work both by having an opioid effect and by enhancing the serotonergic and adrenergic pathways. Its use should be restricted to patients with moderate to severe pain. The dose of tramadol is 50–100 mg 4–6 hourly, depending on the severity of symptoms.

The role of muscle relaxants for back pain remains controversial. A short course of muscle relaxants, such as chlorzoxazone, cyclobenzaprine or carisoprodol, has been found to be more effective than placebo in treating muscle spasm in patients with back pain (Elenbaas, 1980). However, most patients with back pain do not require muscle relaxants and their use should be limited to those patients with marked paravertebral muscle spasm and limited mobility.

Chronic persistent pain with lack of sleep and failed medical or surgical treatment is often associated with psychological and social factors. The usual treatment of physiotherapy and analgesics may not be sufficient to control the symptoms. These patients require a multidisciplinary approach and may need referral to a pain clinic. Some of these patients get good benefit from antidepressants. A short course of a tricylic antidepressant such as amitripty-line at a dose of 25–100 mg at night sometimes also has a secondary analgesic effect and is worth considering in patients with chronic low back pain and disturbed sleep. But it needs to be used in combination with simple analgesia, as on its own it does not have any significant analgesic properties. Antidepressants work slowly and it usually take a few weeks before any clinical improvement is noticed.

Psychotic or opiate analgesics have major limitations for chronic use because of their side-effects, particularly constipation, central nervous system depression and physical dependence.

Role of injection therapy in back pain

Epidural injection

There is no place for routine epidural injection in the management of localized mechanical low back pain. Epidural injections using a mixture of a local anaesthetic and a long-acting corticosteroid have been found to be effective in some patients with nerve root symptoms. However, they should be used only if there is no significant improvement with conservative management, including analgesics and physical modalities.

Both lumbar and caudal sites are used for epidural injection, which can be administered in an outpatient setting. There is a potential for epidural injections to decrease the frequency and intensity of root pain. The usual course of therapy is two to three injections given at intervals of a few days to weeks.

Different studies, however, have produced a mixed result and the role of epidural injection for back pain with root symptoms is still not clear. Those patients with multiple medical problems and those who are a poor surgical risk should, however, be considered for epidural injection. One study has investigated the risk factors that may influence the outcome of lumbar epidural injection. These include low level of education, smoking, lack of employment at the start of treatment, constant pain, sleep disruption, known radicular diagnosis, prolonged duration of pain, change in recreational activities and extreme values on psychogenic scales, and they were associated with failure in univariate analysis. While on logistic regression analysis only prolonged duration, know radicular diagnosis, lack of employment and smoking were significantly associated with increased risk of treatment failure (Hopwood and Abram, 1993).

Facet joint injection

Facet joint pain is usually localized, but it may be referred into the buttocks or down to mid-thigh. Those patients not responding to conservative treatment and those with moderate to severe pain of facet joint origin may be candidates for injection of a local anaesthetic with a long-acting corticosteroid. These injections are given under fluoroscopic control.

Since each facet joint receives a sensory innervation from two spinal levels, i.e. both at and above the level of the involved joint, these injections are given at two sites. Facets injections are usually repeated after 2–4 weeks for a course of two to three injections. The failure rate for facet joint injection is quite high and the improvement in symptoms usually does not last more than 8–12 weeks.

Trigger point injection

In some patients pain is localized to a single spot with associated muscle or ligament tenderness and this may respond to a course of injections of a mixture of a local anaesthetic and a long-acting corticosteroid.

The role of myofascial trigger point injection is not well established. One study found the same beneficial effect with needling the trigger spot with or without medication (Garver, Mark and Wiesel, 1989).

Chemonucleolysis

Chemonucleolysis means intradiscal injection of a proteolytic enzyme. The most commonly used agent is chymopapain. Chemonucleolysis using chymopapain is sometimes used for patients with root symptoms due to a herniated disc.

Proteolytic enzymes such as chymopapain are considered to dissolve the contents of the nucleus pulposus, thereby decreasing pain associated with disc herniation. Chemonucleolysis at present has a limited role in the treatment of low back pain and should be considered only in a very selected group of patients.

References

Assendelft, W.J.J., Koes, B.W. and Knipschild, P.G. *et al.* (1995) The relationship between methodological quality and conclusions in reviews of spinal manipulation. *J. Am. Med. Assoc.*, **274**, 1942–1948.

Bogduk, N. (1992) The sources of low back pain, in *The Lumbar Spine and Back Pain*, 4th edn (ed. M. Tauson), pp. 61–88. Churchill Livingstone, London.

Carey, T.S., Evans, A.T. and Hatler, N.M. *et al.* (1996) Acute severe low back pain: a population base study of prevalence in care seeking. *Spine*, **21**, 339–344.

Damkot, T.K., Pop, M.H., Lord, J. *et al.* (1984) The relationship between work history, work environment and low back pain in men. *Spine*, **9**, 395–399.

Elenbaas, J.K. (1980) Centrally acting oral skeletal muscle relaxants. *Am. J. Hosp. Pharm.*, **37**, 1313–1322.

Frymoyar, J.W. and Cats-Baril, W.L. (1991) An overview of the incidence and cost of low back pain. *Orthop. Clin. N. Am.*, **22**, 363–71.

Garvey, T.E., Mark, M.R. and Wiesel, S.W. (1989) A prospective, randomised, double blinded evaluation of trigger point injections. *Spine*, **14**, 962–964.

Hopwood, M.B. and Abram, S.E. (1993) Factors associated with failure of lumbar epidural steroids. *Reg. Anaesth.*, **18**(4), 238–243.

Papageorgiou, A.C., Croft. P.R., Ferry, S. *et al.* (1995) Estimating the prevalence of low back pain in the general population: evidence from the South Manchester Back Pain Survey. *Spine*, **20**, 1889–1894.

Spitzer, W.O., LeBlabc, F., Dupuis M. *et al.* (1987) Scientific approach to the assessment and management of activity related spinal disorders. *Spine*, **12**, S12-S39.

Osteoporosis

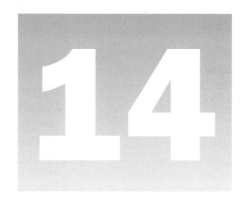

Osteoporosis is very common and affects all races. It is a major public health problem world wide. The prevalence of osteoporosis increases with age and is more common in women than in men, particularly after the menopause. Women, by the age of 50, have a 40% lifetime fracture risk (Cummings *et al.*, 1985). The average age of the population has progressively increased, particularly in the developed world, increasing the prevalence of osteoporosis and its complications.

Bone remodelling is a continuous process characterized by a balanced action of osteoclasts and osteoblasts. Osteoclasts are the cells most important in bone resorption, while osteoblasts are the bone-forming cells. Both these cells are influenced by hormones such as parathyroid hormone, calcitonin, oestrogen and 1,25-dihydroxyvitamin D3.

Osteoporosis is defined as a 'disease characterised by low bone mass and micro-architectural deterioration of bone tissue, leading to enhanced bone fragility and a consequent increase in fracture risk' (Consensus Development Conference, 1993). Normally bone formation and resorption are in equilibrium, while in osteoporosis there is an increased bone resorption compared to bone formation. Bone mineralization is normal, but there is a decrease in total bone mass.

In osteoporosis, bone loss occurs in both the cortical and trabecular areas; trabecular bone loss, however, is predominant in postmenopausal osteoporosis. The main risks for osteoporosis are age and gender, but there are other risk factors and these are listed in Table 14.1.

Symptoms

Generally osteoporosis is silent during its early course and may not produce any symptoms. Some patients develop gradual kyphosis without significant pain. The main symptom of osteoporosis, however, is pain associated with fractures of vertebrae, the wrist or the proximal femur. Multiple fractures are particularly common at the middle and lower part of the thoracic and upper

Table 14.1

Risk factors for osteoporosis

Early menopause
Hysterectomy
Long-term or large doses of corticosteroids
Hypogonadism
Family history of osteoporosis
Alcohol abuse
Thyrotoxicosis
Malabsorption/malnutrition
Chronic renal failure
Chronic liver failure
Rheumatoid arthritis

part of the lumbar spine and their frequency increases with age (Bengner, Johnell and Redlund-Johnell, 1988).

In many patients, particularly the elderly, osteoporotic fractures may not receive any clinical attention. Generally, however, vertebral fractures present with acute thoracic or back pain of sudden onset brought on by minimal effort, such as bending or lifting.

Fracture of the wrist usually occurs after falling forwards on to an outstretched hand, while hip fractures commonly occur when falling backwards or on to the side. In the majority of patients a fracture at the hip is brought on by a fall, though there is some evidence that pain may be the initial symptom leading to the fall (Maugers *et al.*, 1996). However, fracture of the proximal femur can occur spontaneously, without any preceding history of trauma (Dorne and Lander, 1985). The other fractures associated with osteoporosis which may cause pain are rib fractures. These more commonly occur in patients on long-term corticosteroids and those with Cushing's syndrome.

The intensity of pain associated with a vertebral fracture is variable, but is usually described by patients as a severe sharp pain followed a few days later by a dull nagging pain. It diminishes significantly 4–6 weeks after onset.

Generally the pain associated with a lumbar osteoporotic fracture does not radiate into the legs and very rarely produces neurological symptoms. Some patients have difficulty in sleeping on their back and the pain is also made worse on prolonged standing, forward flexion or backward extension and on lifting and carrying weight.

Physical examination findings usually depend on the severity of osteoporosis and the area predominantly effected by the condition or its complications. In well-established spinal osteoporosis there is thoracic kyphosis and loss of height. With the passage of time the abdomen becomes more prominent. Those presenting with acute vertebral collapse are very tender overlying the corresponding vertebra, with paravertebral muscle spasm and restricted, painful spinal movements.

Management

The three important goals in the management of osteoporosis and associated complications are:

1. to prevent further bone loss;
2. to alleviate pain;
3. rehabilitation.

This section will only deal with treatment of pain in association with osteoporosis, particularly the pain of osteoporotic vertebral collapse, as generally patients with wrist and hip fractures are treated surgically.

The main pharmacological treatments of osteoporosis are outlined in Table 14.2 and will not be discussed any further.

The management of osteoporotic vertebral collapse is multidisciplinary and should be individualized depending on the needs of the patient. A vertebral fracture can present in three ways:

- asymptomatic vertebral fracture
- acute vertebral fracture
- chronic pain due to vertebral fracture.

Table 14.2
Pharmacological agents used in the treatment of osteoporosis

Antiresorptive agents
  Oestrogens
  Calcium
  Vitamin D
  Bisphosphonates
  Calcitonin
  Thiazides

Bone-stimulating/formation agents
  Sodium fluoride
  Combined pill (oestrogen, progestin and androgens)
  Vitamin D metabolites
  Anabolic steroids

A small minority of patients with an osteoporotic vertebral fracture may be asymptomatic and may just present with long-standing kyphosis. Osteoporotic fractures occur more commonly in elderly patients, who also are more prone to pain due to degenerative disease of the spine and peripheral osteoarthritis and may not present with acute pain as many consider pain to be part and parcel of growing old. Management goals for these patients include secondary prevention of osteoporosis with pharmacological agents and, most importantly, a rehabilitation programme including advice regarding diet, exercise and mobility to prevent new fractures.

For those presenting with acute or chronic pain the initial treatment should be directed at the pain. Many patients believe that the pain and disability associated with these fractures could be permanent and it is therefore prudent to explain the diagnosis and prognosis to these patients at the onset. The drugs most commonly used for the management of the pain are summarized in Table 14.3.

During the acute stage, the pain is localized over the vertebral fracture and is made worse by movement. Patients should therefore be advised bed rest for a few days to minimize this. Simple painkillers, such as paracetamol, are usually inadequate to control the pain and the majority of patients require stronger analgesia, such as codeine or tramadol on a regular basis. A small minority of patients may require regular morphine or pethidine for 3–4 days, followed by dihydrocodeine or tramadol. Narcotic analgesics are good at controlling pain but have to be used with caution in elderly patients, who are more prone to their side-effects, particularly drowsiness and hence falls leading to further fractures. Epidural injections for pain relief have been tried in vertebral osteoporotic fractures (Waldman and Greek, 1994), but generally there is no evidence that epidural injections help.

Non-steroidal anti-inflammatory drugs (NSAIDs) do not usually have a role to play for painful acute or chronic vertebral fractures. Further management of pain after the initial week depends on the severity of pain and degree of osteoporosis. Patients should be encouraged to mobilize as

Table 14.3
Drugs used for the management of pain in vertebral fracture

Narcotics
Codeine or dihydrocodeine
Tramadol
Morphine and pethidine (only in very severe cases and for a short period)
Calcitonin
intranasal
intramuscular

soon as possible. If persistent pain is restricting mobility, some patients may be helped by the use of an orthosis. Different types of support devices, including bracing and lightweight external supports for the lumbar spine, may be helpful during the acute stage (Jurisson, 1991). Their prolonged use should be discouraged.

Calcitonin is licensed for use in established osteoporosis, but is also used for the treatment of pain due to vertebral osteoporotic fractures. It has been used both intranasally and intramuscularly with good effect. The intranasal route of administration appears to give better analgesic effect than the intramuscular route (Pun and Chan, 1989; Gennari, Agnusdei and Camporeale, 1991; Pontiorli *et al.*, 1991). Its analgesic effect appears to be unrelated to its antiresorptive bone effect. The exact mechanism of the analgesic effect of calcitonin is not known (Kapuscinski *et al.*, 1996).

Since there is some evidence that androgenic steroids may stimulate osteoblasts, one study compared the effects of an androgenic steroid nandrolone decanoate, with that of a vitamin metabolite in a group of postmenopausal women with osteoporotic fracture and found significantly better pain control in the group taking nandrolone (Lyritis *et al.*, 1989). These compounds, however, are not used routinely for the management of chronic pain due to vertebral collapse.

Unlike hip and distal forearm fractures, surgery has a very limited role to play in the management of acute or chronic pain in vertebral osteoporotic fractures. A small group of patients may develop neurological complications secondary to vertebral fracture or the spine may become unstable and require surgery. In one small study of four patients vertebral fracture vertebroplasty was effective in relieving back pain (Gangi, Kastler and Dietemann, 1994). A recent article has reviewed this aspect of management of vertebral collapse in detail (Chiras *et al.*, 1997).

Physiotherapy is an important aspect of treatment in this group during the acute and chronic stages. During the acute stage physiotherapy modalities, including ice and heat massage, are often very helpful in diminishing the intensity of pain. Long-term rehabilitation programmes to promote bone mass and improve mobility with regular exercises, and advice to improve posture and muscle strength and to relief pain are important adjuncts to the pharmacological treatment (Rudd, 1989).

References

Bengner, U., Johnell, O. and Redlund-Johnell, I. (1988) Changes in incidence and prevalence of vertebral fractures during 30 years. *Cal. Tis. Int.*, **42**, 293–296.

Chiras, J., Depriester, C., Weill, A. *et al.* (1997) Percutaneous vertebral surgery. Techniques and indications. Vertebroplasties percutaneous. Technique et indications. *J. Neuroradiol.*, **24**(1), 45–59.

Consensus Development Conference (1993) Diagnosis, prophylaxis, and treatment of osteoporosis. *Am. J. Med.*, **94**, 646–650.

Cummings, S.R., Kelsey, J.L., Nevitt, M.C. *et al.* (1985) Epidemiology of osteoporosis and osteoporotic fractures. *Epidemiol. Rev.*, 7, 178–208.

Dorne, H.L, and Lander, B.H. (1985) Spontaneous stress fractures of the femoral neck. *Am. J. Roentgenol.*, **144**(2), 343–347.

Gangi, A., Kastler, B.A. and Dietemann, J.L. (1994) Percutaneous vertebroplasty guided by a combination of CT and fluoroscopy. *Am. J. Neuroradiol.*, **15**, 83–86.

Gennari, C., Agnusdei, D. and Camporeale, A. (1991) Use of calcitonin in the treatment of bone pain associated with osteoporosis. *Cal. Tis. Int.*, **49**, Suppl. 2, S9–S13.

Jurisson, M.L. (1991) Rehabilitation in rheumatic diseases. What's new. *W. J. Med.*, **154**(5), 545–548.

Kapuscinski, P., Talalaj, M., Borowicz, J. *et al.* (1996). An analgesic effect of synthetic human calcitonin in patients with primary osteoporosis. *Mat. Med. Pol.*, **28**(3), 83–86.

Lyritis, G.P., Mayasis, B., Tsakalakos, N. *et al.* (1989) The natural history of the osteoporotic vertebral fracture. *Clin. Rheumatol.*, **8**, Suppl. 2, 66–69.

Maugars, Y., Dubois, F., Berthelot, J.M. *et al.* (1996) Pain due to bone insufficiency as a symptom heralding femoral neck fracture. *Rev. Rhum.* (English edn), **63**(1), 30–35.

Pontiorli, A.E., Pajetta, E., Calderara, A. *et al.* (1991) Intranasal and intramuscular human calcitonin in female osteoporosis and Paget's disease of bones: a pilot study. *J. Endocrinol. Invest.*, **14**, 47–51.

Pun, K.K. and Chan, L.W. (1989) Analgesic effect of intranasal salmon calcitonin in the treatment of osteoporotic vertebral fractures. *Clin. Therapeut.*, **11**(2), 205–209.

Rudd, E. (1989) Preventive aspects of mobility and functional disability. *Scand. J. Rheumatol.*, Suppl., **82**, 25–32.

Waldman, S.D. and Greek, C.R. (1994) Compression fractures: consider epidural nerve blocks for pain relief. *Geriatrics*, **49**(7), 15.

Paget's disease

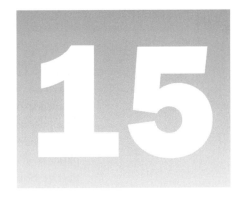

Paget's disease is a localized bone disorder characterized by an abnormal increase in bone formation and remodelling. Its prevalence increases after the age of 40, when in the UK it is about 3.6%, and it approximately doubles for each decade from the age of 50 (Kanis, 1991). It is more common in men than women in a ratio of about 3:2. The distribution of Paget's disease is world wide, but its prevalence is low in the Middle East, Africa and Asia.

Pathophysiology

The exact aetiology of Paget's disease is unknown, however various theories have been put forward. It is characterized by increased osteoblastic activity, resulting in resorption of bone at a particular site followed by an increase in new bone formation. The compensatory increase in new bone formation, however, is disorganized and results in localized enlargement. The newly formed bone is abnormal both macro- and microscopically, is more fragile and is prone to spontaneous fracture.

Clinical features

During its early course Paget's disease is usually asymptomatic. As the disease progresses it may manifest itself in various ways, including localized bony deformity, localized bone pain and pain due osteoarthritis, neurological complications, spontaneous fracture, cardiovascular complications and, rarely, malignant transformation.

BONE AND JOINTS

A large proportion of patients with Paget's disease remain asymptomatic. Localized pain, however, is the presenting complaint in about 80% of patients. The sites most commonly affected are the pelvis, spine, long bones and base of the skull. Sometimes Paget's may present with bone pain localized to ankle (Neylon, 1995), heel (Lichniak, 1990) or scapula (Ueda *et al.*, 1996).

The pain of Paget's disease is usually deep seated and diffuse. Many patients also complain of joint pain at sites near the abnormally formed pagetic bone. The deformities of the limb bones cause mechanical stress on the joints and can lead to osteoarthritis with associated features. The most common sites are the hip and knee. Vertebral involvement leads to enlargement which may in turn lead to entrapment neuropathy and, rarely, cauda equina syndrome.

The Paget's bone is fragile and can fracture following minor trauma or spontaneously. Fractures most commonly occur at right angles to the long axis of the weight-bearing long bones such as the femur and tibia.

Malignant transformation occurs very rarely. Males above the age of 50 are most commonly affected, with the femur as the major site. The most common malignant tumour transformation is to osteosarcoma, but other forms such as chondrosarcoma and fibrosarcoma can also occur. Worsening localized pain and a palpable mass should raise concern. Prognosis in these cases is rather poor.

NEUROLOGICAL COMPLICATIONS

These are usually a consequence of the localized bone enlargement. In the skull this can lead to entrapment neuropathies of the second, fifth, seventh and eighth cranial nerves, as these nerves pass through the bony foramina. Other complications include diminished vision and blindness due to pressure on the optic nerve and deafness due to the compression of the auditory canal. When the base of the skull is enlarged it can lead to vertebro basilar vascular insufficiency or brainstem compression and hydro-cephalus.

Spinal vertebral enlargement can lead to vertebral collapse and may cause nerve entrapment or cauda equina syndrome.

VASCULAR COMPLICATIONS

Pagetic bone is highly vascular. This increased vascularity has both a local and systemic effect. The local effect is usually an increase in the overlying skin temperature. The increased peripheral blood flow increases cardiac output and can lead to high-output cardiac failure in susceptible in-dividuals. The increased blood flow to the pagetic bone in the skull can be at the expense of blood supply to the brain, causing central nervous system side-effects of ischaemia.

Investigations

In Paget's disease there is a high bone turnover and this leads to increased production of alkaline phosphatase and osteocalcin. The other marker of pagetic activity includes urinary excretion of total hydroxyproline and pyridinoline.

The plain X-ray findings in well-established Paget's are quite characteristic and include localized expansion of bone with an abnormal trabecular pattern. The isotope bone scan with 99-technetium-labelled bisphosphonate is very helpful in diagnosis. Bone biopsy is generally not required to establish the diagnosis.

Treatment

There are three major aspects to the management of Paget's disease:

- pain control
- prevention of fractures and other complications
- avoidance minimization of disfigurement.

ANALGESICS

The intensity of pain in Paget's disease varies widely. It can be localized or referred due to nerve entrapment. The initial management is usually with a combination of a simple analgesic and a non-steroidal anti-inflammatory drug (NSAID). Depending on the severity of the pain, the patient may require paracetamol, codeine or tramadol. Since most patients with Paget's disease are elderly, one has to use NSAIDs with caution to avoid serious side-effects. The role of analgesics and NSAIDs is purely symptomatic. These agents have no effect on the progression of disease or the prognosis.

ANTIOSTEOCLASTIC AGENTS

The agents most widely used are:

- bisphosphonates
- calcitonin.

Table 15.1
Currently available
bisphosphonates

Category	Name
First generation	etidronate
Second generation	clodronate
	pamidronate
Third generation	tiludronate
	alendronate
	risedronate

Both bisphosphonates and calcitonin are antiosteoclastic agents and therefore reduce the remodelling activity. This results in a decrease in bone pain and an improvement of radiological appearances (Gutteridge *et al.*, 1996; Siris *et al.*, 1996). However, this may take a long time. These agents also improve the biochemical markers, including a fall in serum alkaline phosphatase, and urinary markers.

Relapses occur following remission particularly after calcitonin use. For monitoring it is advisable to check bone markers twice a year.

Calcitonin has been used extensively for the treatment of Paget's disease and is very effective in relieving bone pain. It is available in a nasal spray and in suppository form, as well as parenterally. Since in most cases, after long use, it is unable to suppress the bone turnover by more than 50%, bisphosphonates are increasingly being used for the treatment of Paget's disease.

Several bisphosphonates are available (Table.15.1). Some of the new bisphosphonates are still undergoing trials, while others have been used successfully for quite some time. The latter include etidronate, the use of which has declined for various reasons. The new second-generation compounds which are being increasingly used include disodium pamidronate, clodronate, alendronate and risedronate.

References

Gutteridge, D.H., Retallack, R.W., Ward, L.C. *et al.* (1996). Clinical, biochemical, hematologic, and radiographic responses in Paget's disease following intravenous pamidronate disodium: a 2-year study. *Bone*, **19**(4), 387–394.

Kanis, J.A. (1991) *Pathophysiology and Treatment of Paget's Disease of Bone*, Martin Dunitz, London.

Lichniak, J.E. (1990) The heel in systemic disease. *Clin. Pod. Med.*, 7(2), 225–241.

Neylon, T.A. (1995) Paget's disease of bone presenting as chronic ankle pain. *J. Am. Pod. Med. Assoc.*, **85**(10), 556–559.

Siris, E., Weinstein, R.S., Altman, R. *et al.* (1996) Comparative study of alendronate versus etidronate for the treatment of Paget's disease of bone. *J. Clin. Endocrinol.*, **81**(3), 961–967.

Ueda, T., Healey, J.H., Huvos A.G. and Panicek, D.M. (1996) Scapular pain and swelling in a 60-year-old man with Paget's disease. *Clin. Orthopaed. Rel. Res.*, **326**, 284–286, 310–312.

Ankylosing spondylitis

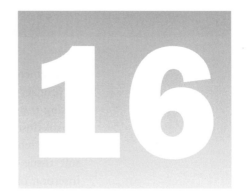

Ankylosing spondylitis is a chronic systemic inflammatory condition that mainly effects the sacroiliac joints and the spine, and less commonly involves the peripheral joints. Its name is derived from the Greek words *angkylos* meaning 'bent' and *spondylos* meaning 'spinal vertebra'.

For classification purposes ankylosing spondylitis is included in the group of diseases labelled seronegative spondyloarthropathy. The other members include Reiter's syndrome, reactive arthritis, psoriatic arthritis, arthritis associated with inflammatory bowel disease, such as Crohn's, ulcerative colitis and Whipple's disease.

Clinical features

Ankylosing spondylitis usually starts at an earlier age, the average age of onset being approximately 26 years. It is rare for it to start after the age of 40. Ankylosing spondylitis is three times more common in men than women. The annual incidence among American whites is 6.6 cases per 1 000 000 people (Carter *et al.*, 1979). However, the prevalence of ankylosing spondylitis among the black population is very low.

The back pain of ankylosing spondylitis has certain special features differentiating it from mechanical low back pain (Brown, 1989). It is usually of slow onset and the intensity varies from a mild ache to severe pain made worse on coughing or sneezing. The pain is felt deep to the gluteal region over the lower lumbar area. Low back pain with stiffness is the hallmark of ankylosing spondylitis and is the initial symptom in about 75% of patients. Low back pain of inflammatory origin usually improves with exercise.

The initial involvement in ankylosing spondylitis is usually of the sacroiliac joint and can be unilateral or bilateral. The back pain and stiffness is worse in the morning and after inactivity. These symptoms usually improve by taking a hot shower in the morning or after gentle exercise. Ankylosing spondylitis rarely involves the hip and shoulder joints, and the involvement of more peripheral joints, e.g. the knee and ankle, is infrequent in primary ankylosing spondylitis. Some patients present with chest pain arising from the thoracic spine, costosternal or costovertebral areas.

Ankylosing spondylitis symptoms are predominantly from axial and to a lesser extent from peripheral arthritis, but sometimes they may be due to soft tissue lesions, i.e. enthesitis. There are inflammatory changes at the insertion of tendons, ligaments or articular capsule into bone, e.g. Achilles tendonitis. Enthesitis may be the initial manifestation of the ankylosing spondylitis. The main symptom is pain and there may or may not be associated swelling at the insertion site.

Ankylosing spondylitis is a multisystem disease with extra-articular manifestations, including pulmonary and cardiovascular involvement, acute anterior uveitis, and amyloidosis.

Investigations

In well-established ankylosing spondylitis the diagnosis can be made by just observing the patient's spine with its characteristic posture. However, in the early stages the diagnosis is sometimes not easy to make by examination alone and one has to rely on further investigations.

The biochemical test, including ESR and CRP, may be elevated in ankylosing spondylitis; however, these inflammatory markers do not necessarily correlate with clinical disease activity (Kahn and Kushner, 1984). About 15% of patients with ankylosing spondylitis have mild normochromic, normocytic anaemia.

Radiological changes, however, are the hallmark of ankylosing spondylitis, especially in the sacroiliac joints. The radiographic changes in the sacroiliac joints, are usually symmetrical, but could involve one joint more than the other. These changes consist of blurring of the subchondral bone, followed by sclerosis of the adjacent bone with erosions. The inflammatory changes in the spine lead to fusion in the facet joints and ossification of the spinal ligaments, with squaring of the vertebral bodies. These changes progress gradually to complete fusion of the vertebral column, i.e. bamboo spine.

There is a strong association of HLA B27 with ankylosing spondylitis. About 90–95% of patients with ankylosing spondylitis are HLA B27 positive. There is, however, wide racial and ethnic variation in the prevalence of HLA B27. HLA B27 is almost non-existent in African blacks while in Papua New Guinea its prevalence is about 52% (Khan, 1987; Bhatia *et al.*, 1988).

Management

A multidisciplinary approach is the best way to manage ankylosing spondylitis. The usual team members are physiotherapists, occupational therapists, chiropodists, social workers, physicians and, rarely, surgeons. Accordingly the management of ankylosing spondylitis can be divided into three:

- non-pharmacological
- pharmacological
- surgical.

NON-PHARMACOLOGICAL

Ankylosing spondylitis is a chronic progressive condition leading to stiffening and fusion of the spine and peripheral joints. Early recognition and patient education are the most important aspects of management. The initial aims of management are to reduce pain and stiffness and to restore and maintain posture and mobility.

Regular physiotherapy is the single most important aspect of management. Patients should initially be taught exercises to mobilize the spine and then encouraged to maintain an exercise programme at home with regular 3–6 monthly visits to the physiotherapy department to assess progress. Measurement of movements, particularly of the spine, i.e. cervical, lumbar and chest expansion, should be done at the initial visit and then at 6–12 months intervals.

PHARMACOLOGICAL

The pharmacological agents used in the treatment of ankylosing spondylitis include:

- simple analgesics
- non-steroidal anti-inflammatory drugs
- second-line disease-modifying agents
- corticosteroids.

The pain and stiffness in the majority of patients with ankylosing spondylitis is controlled with regular physiotherapy and judicious use of a non-steroidal anti-inflammatory drug (NSAID).

Almost all NSAIDs have some role to play in the management of ankylosing spondylitis. However, they usually need to be given in relatively high doses. In the past indomethacin was the most widely used NSAID. But other commonly prescribed NSAIDs, such as nabumetone (Palferman and

Webley, 1991), diclofenac (Calabro, 1986), and flurbiprofen (Lomen *et al.*, 1986) are also very effective when compared to indomethacin.

The use of phenylbutazone has declined over the years. In the UK phenylbutazone may be prescribed only by hospital consultants on a named patient basis. Phenylbutazone is considered to inhibit the calcification of syndesmophyte (Boersma, 1976). It has also been suggested that indomethacin slows the radiological progression of ankylosing spondylitis (Lehdinen, 1979). NSAID have no direct effect on the prognosis. However, by decreasing pain and stiffness, they allow the patient to adhere to a regular exercise programme which is the most important aspect of treatment.

Second-line disease-modifying drugs have also been used in the treatment of ankylosing spondylitis. Almost all those used in the treatment of rheumatoid arthritis have also been used in ankylosing spondylitis with variable effect. Sulphasalazine is the most commonly prescribed second-line drug in ankylosing spondylitis for spinal and peripheral joint disease and has had mixed results (Corkill *et al.*, 1990; Ferraz *et al.*, 1990). In a small study olsalazine was found to be effective in patients unresponsive to NSAIDs and physiotherapy (Chapman and Zwillich, 1994). Methotrexate has recently been increasingly used in patients with ankylosing spondylitis with mixed results (Creemers *et al.*, 1995). The usual starting dose is 7.5–15 mg weekly. In one small study rifampin SV was given to patients with ankylosing spondylitis and produced a significant reduction in inflammatory markers and painful joints (Caruso, Cazzola and Santandrea, 1992).

Local corticosteroid injections into the sacroiliac joint have been evaluated in a double-blind study which showed a significant clinical improvement in the corticosteroid injected group (Maugars *et al.*, 1996). Local corticosteroid injection into the sacroiliac joint is not an easy technique; it has to be carried out under an image intensifier.

Regular oral corticosteroids are generally not used in the treatment of ankylosing spondylitis. One study, however, has compared the effect of three consecutive days of high- (1000 mg) and low-dose (375 mg) methylprednisolone infusions. There was no placebo group. Improvement in pain relief and mobility was observed in both groups, with the high-dose group yielding a greater and prolonged improvement (Peters and Ejstrup, 1992). In another study methylprednisolone infusions were also found to be beneficial in patients with active ankylosing spondylitis (Ejstrup and Peters, 1985). However, methylprednisolone infusions should be restricted to patients with active ankylosing spondylitis not responding to NSAIDs or in those where NSAIDs are contraindicated.

Soft-tissue lesions such as Achilles enthesitis and tendonitis can be difficult to treat. In some patients the stringent treatment, including physiotherapy, orthotic devices and anti-inflammatory drugs, is not helpful. The role of local corticosteroid injections for an inflamed Achilles tendon is controversial because of the possibility of subsequent tendon rupture. Those patients with persistent severe plantar fasciitis not responding to conservative treatment may benefit from a trial of local radiotherapy (Mantel, 1978).

Surgery has an important role in patients with atlanto-axial subluxation and in patients with a painful hip due to advanced arthritis.

References

Bhatia, K., Parasad, M.L., Darnish, G. *et al.* (1988) Antigen and heplotype frequencies at 3 human leucocyte antigen (HLA - A, - B, -C) in the Pawaia of Papua New Guinea. *Am. J. Phys. Anthropol.*, **75**, 329–340.

Boersma, J.W. (1976) Retardation of ossification of the lumbar vertebral column in ankylosing spondylitis by means of phenylbutazone. *Scand. J. Rheumatol.*, **5**, 60–64.

Brown, M.D. (1989) The source of low back pain. *Semin. Arthritis Rheum.*, **18**, Suppl. 2 67–72.

Calabro, J.J. (1986) Efficacy of diclofenac in ankylosing spondylitis. *Am. J. Med.*, **80**(4B), 58–63.

Carter, E.T., McKenna, C.H., Bryan D.D. *et al.* (1979) Epidemiology of ankylosing spondylitis in Rochester, Minnesota 1935–73. *Arthritis Rheum.*, **25**, 365–370.

Caruso, I., Cazzola, M. and Santandrea, S. (1992) Clinical improvement in ankylosing spondylitis with rifamycin SV infiltrations of peripheral joints. *J. Int. Med. Res.*, **20**(2), 171–181.

Chapman, C.M. and Zwillich, S.H. (1994) Olsalazine in ankylosing spondylitis: a pilot study. *J. Rheumatol.*, **21**(9), 1699–1701.

Corkill, M.M., Jobanputra, P., Gibson, T. and Macfarlane D.G. (1990) A controlled trial of sulphasalazine treatment of chronic ankylosing spondylitis: failure to demonstrate a clinical effect. *Br. J. Rheumatol.*, **29**(1), 41–45.

Creemers, M.C., Franssen, M.J., Van De Putte, L.B. *et al.* (1995) Methotrexate in severe ankylosing spondylitis, an open study. *J. Rheumatol.*, **22**(6), 1104–1107.

Ejstrup, L. and Peters, N.D. (1985) Intravenous methylprednisolone pulse therapy in ankylosing spondylitis. *Dan. Med. Bull.*, **32**(4), 231–233.

Ferraz, M.B., Tugwell, P., Goldsmith C.H. and Atra, E. (1990) Meta-analysis of sulfasalazine in ankylosing spondylitis. *J. Rheumatol.*, **17**(11), 1482–1486.

Khan, M.A. (1987) HLA and ankylosing spondylitis, in *Ankylosing Spondylitis. New Clinical Applications. Rheumatology* (eds J.J. Calabro and Carson-Dicks), MTP, England, pp.23–44.

Kahn, M.A. and Kushner, I. (1984) Diagnosis of ankylosing spondylitis, in *Progress in Clinical Rheumatology*, vol. 1, (ed. A.S. Cohen), pp. 145–178. Giune and Stratton, Orlando.

Lehdinen, R. (1979) Clinical and radiological features of ankylosing spondylitis in the 1950's and 1976 in the same hospital. *Scand. J. Rheumatol.*, **8**: 57–61.

Lomen, P.L., Turner, L.F., Lamborn, K.R. and Brinn, E.L. (1986) Flurbiprofen in the treatment of ankylosing spondylitis. A comparison with indomethacin. *Am. J. Med.*, **80**(3A), 127–132.

Mantel, B.S. (1978) Radiotherapy for painful heel syndrome. *Br. Med. J.*, **2**, 90–91.

Maugars, Y., Mathis, C., Berthelot, J.M. *et al.* (1996) Assessment of the efficacy of sacro iliac corticosteroid injections in spondyloarthropathies, a double blind study. *Br. J. Rheumatol.*, **35**(8): 767–770.

Palferman, T.G. and Webley, M.A. (1991) comparative study of nabumetone and indomethacin in ankylosing spondylitis. *Europ. J. Rheumatol. Inflam.*, **11**(2) 23–29.

Peters, N.D. and Ejstrup, L. (1992) Intravenous methylprednisolone pulse therapy in ankylosing spondylitis. *Scand. J. Rheumatol.*, **21**(3), 134–138.

Reflex sympathetic dystrophy

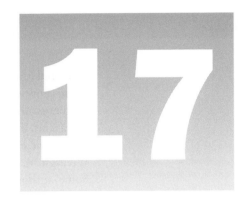

Reflex sympathetic dystrophy is a complex condition first described as a complication of traumatic injuries in the American Civil War (Mitchell, Morehouse and Keen, 1864). There is still considerable disagreement to its aetiology, management and even on what to call it. There is a plethora of synonyms, including algodystrophy, Sudeck's atrophy, causalgia and shoulder–hand syndrome. Generally, for those writing in English, the term reflex sympathetic dystrophy is preferred, those writing in French prefer the term algodystrophy and the Germans use Sudeck's atrophy. However, the International Association for the Study of Pain recently classified 'reflex sympathetic dystrophy' and 'causalgia' as Regional Pain Syndrome I and II (Walker and Cousins, 1997).

Epidemiology

The epidemiology of reflex sympathetic dystrophy is poorly defined, mainly because of a lack of diagnostic criteria. The condition, however, occurs world wide and affects every race. It is seen more commonly between 40 and 60 years of age, but also occurs in children and the elderly. In children, girls are more affected than boys.

There is a strong association with trauma, Colles' fracture and in patients with hemiplegia. It has also been reported following shingles and myocardial infarction.

Aetiology

The exact aetiology of this rather complex condition is unknown. However, various theories have been put forward to explain abnormalities at the peripheral, spinal and supraspinal level (Hardy and Hardy, 1997). The peripheral changes include initial vasomotor reflex spasm leading to a loss of vascular tone, which causes vasodilation and local bone resorption. It is suggested that impaired mobility then leads to a further decrease in local blood flow which eventually leads to the fibrosis and shortening of the ligaments on the affected site (Poplawski, Wiley and Murray, 1983).

Various theories have been put forward to explain these local abnormal vasomotor changes, including abnormalities of the central nervous system (Livingston, 1947) and peripheral nervous system (Hooshmand, 1993). Some authors have suggested psychological disturbance as a major predisposing factor (Egle and Hoffman, 1990; Van Houdenhove *et al.*, 1992).

Clinical features

Reflex sympathetic dystrophy is a complex condition with variable presentations. The cardinal symptoms, however, are severe localized pain associated with swelling and autonomic vasomotor dysfunction associated with impaired mobility. This may be associated with trophic skin changes and impaired ability of the involved part.

The pain in reflex sympathetic dystrophy is usually diffuse and affects an extremity. There is usually an associated allodynia. Patients usually describe a severe 'burning' or 'bursting' pain. The signs of autonomic vasomotor disturbance usually include a very sensitive skin to superficial and deep pressure and even to temperature changes. There is usually a bluish tint of the involved skin. The localized skin temperature is usually higher initially and later on the affected part becomes cold, which may or may not be associated with sweating. In some patients the nails become brittle and there is excessive growth of hair. The chronic untreated condition can lead to contractures.

Reflex sympathetic dystrophy usually has three distinct clinical stages. There is, however, considerable overlap and in many patients there is no distinct transition from stage 1 to stage 3. In stage 1 there is usually severe pain, allodynia, swelling and vasomotor changes. X-rays show diffuse osteopaenia of the involved part. In the second stage the pain persists, but in addition there are atrophic skin changes, including cyanosis, coldness and stiffness of the area involved. Stage 3 is the advanced stage of skin and subcutaneous tissue atrophy with associated contractures. In stage 3 there may or may not be any localized pain.

Investigation

There has been no consistently abnormal finding in the haematological or biochemical parameters of these patients. Some studies, however, have found an increase in urinary hydroxyproline excretion, whilst others have reported a marginal increase in serum alkaline phosphatase and osteocalcin activity.

A plain radiograph in the early stages is usually not much help, as radiological changes may take several weeks or even months to appear. It is important to note that in some patients radiological changes may never appear, and therefore X-ray findings are not diagnostic. However, in some patients there is a varying degree of homogeneous or heterogeneous bone demineralization. Sometimes these changes are very mild and it is therefore important to compare the corresponding side of the opposite limb with a similar radiological view.

A radioisotope bone scan may be helpful in diagnosis. In patients with reflex sympathetic dystrophy there is usually a characteristic delayed bone scan pattern involving the affected part.

The other methods used to detect these localized changes include tomodensitometry, vascular scintography, thermography and local magnetic resonance imagining.

Management

It is very important to start treatment as soon as the diagnosis has been established, since there is evidence that early therapeutic intervention results in a better outcome. The intensity of the pain in reflex sympathetic dystrophy is usually severe and simple analgesics, including non-steroidal anti-inflammatory drugs (NSAIDs) are of limited use, but can be very effective in a minority of patients. It is imperative to explain the diagnosis and prognosis to patients. The management of reflex sympathetic dystrophy is multidisciplinary, involving patient, family physician and a specialist with an interest in this condition.

There are no well-controlled studies on the use of antidepressants, transcutaneous electric nerve stimulation, acupuncture or psychotherapy in the treatment of reflex sympathetic dystrophy. Nevertheless, these modalities are sometimes helpful in complicated cases (Fialka *et al.*, 1993). Corticosteroids in the dose of 30–40 mg daily in the initial 4–6 weeks have been found to be helpful by some authors (Kozin *et al.*, 1976), while others have used long-acting intramuscular corticosteroids with mixed results (Grundberg, 1996).

Calcitonin in widely used for the treatment of pain relief. It is used both intramuscularly and subcutaneously or intranasaly (Mundun *et al.*, 1993; Hamamci *et al.*, 1996). The usual dose is 100–160 IU daily for 4–6 weeks followed by an injection every other day for about 3–6 weeks (Gobelat, Waldburger and Meier, 1992).

Sympathetic blockade in the form of a regional guanethidine block is widely used with mixed results. There is a place for this form of treatment for short-term relief in a selected group of patients (Field and Atkins, 1993; Field, Monk and Atkins, 1993). However, long-term results have been rather disappointing (Ramamurthy and Hoffman, 1995; Kaplan *et al.*, 1996). One study has reported good outcome by using a combination of ketorolac–lidocaine regional anaesthesia (Connelly, Reuben and Brull, 1995). If, however, there is no improvement with a series of blocks in a selected group of patients, then chemical or surgical sympathectomy is worth a trial.

Recently there have been a few reports of successful treatment of pain and swelling with bisphosphonates (Adami *et al.*, 1997; Cortet *et al.*, 1997). The improvement in pain, swelling and range of motion has been attributed to the prevention of bone resorption with bisphosphonates. There have also been reports of successful treatment of reflex sympathetic dystrophy with intrathecal morphine (Becker *et al.*, 1995), subarachnoid clonidine (Kabeer and Hardy, 1996), oral nifedipine and alpha-sympathetic blocker phenoxy-benzamine (Muizelaar *et al.*, 1997), topical nitroglycerin (Manahan *et al.*, 1993) and electroconvulsive therapy (King and Nuss, 1993). Gabapentine, which is a relatively new anticonvulsant, was used successfully in six patients with severe and refractory reflex sympathetic dystrophy (Mellick and Mellick, 1997). Severe cases not responding to the conventional treatment may respond to the regular use of a spinal cord stimulator implant (Kumar, Nath and Toth, 1997). This is an expensive device with very few complications reported so far. It is, however, only available in specialized centres.

The long-term prognosis in reflex sympathetic dystrophy is variable. If untreated, it has the potential to lead to severe physical disabilities. Therefore it is very important to recognize the condition early on and to treat its symptoms in a multidisciplinary team approach.

References

Adami, S., Fossaluzza, V., Gatti, D. *et al.* (1997) Bisphosphonate therapy of reflex sympathetic dystrophy syndrome. *Ann. Rheum. Dis.*, **56**(3), 201–204.

Becker, W.J., Ablett, D.P., Harris, C.J. and Dold, O.N. (1995) Long term treatment of intractable reflex sympathetic dystrophy with intrathecal morphine. *Can. J. Neurol. Sci.*, **22**(2), 153–159.

Connelly, N.R., Reuben, S. and Brull, S.J. (1995) Intravenous regional anesthesia with ketorolac–lidocaine for the management of sympathetically-mediated pain. *Yale J. Bio. Med.*, **68**(3–4), 95–99.

Cortet, B., Flipo, R.M., Coquerelle, P. *et al.* (1997) Treatment of severe, recalcitrant reflex sympathetic dystrophy: assessment of efficacy and safety of the second generation bisphosphonate Pamidronate. *Clin. Rheumatol.*, **16**(1), 51–56.

Egle, U.T. and Hoffman, S.O. (1990) Psychosomatic correlations of sympathetic reflex dystrophy (Sudeck's disease). Review of the literature and initial clinical results. *Psychother. Psychosom. Med. Psychol.*, **40**, 123–135.

Fialka, V., Resch, K.L., Ritter-Dietrich, D. *et al.* (1993) Acupuncture for reflex sympathetic dystrophy. *Arch. Int. Med.*, **153**(5), 661, 665.

Field, J. and Atkins, R.M. (1993) Effect of guanethidine on the natural history of post-traumatic algodystrophy. *Ann. Rheum. Dis.*, **52**(6), 467–469.

Field, J., Monk, C. and Atkins, R.M. (1993) Objective improvements in algodystrophy following regional intravenous guanethidine. *J. Hand Surg.* (Brit. vol.), **18**(3), 339–342.

Gobelat, C., Waldburger, M. and Meier, J.L. (1992) The effect of adding calcitonin to physical treatment on reflex sympathetic dystrophy. *Pain*, **48**, 171–175.

Grundberg, A.B. (1996) Reflex sympathetic dystrophy: treatment with long-acting intramuscular corticosteroids. *J. Hand Surg.* (Am. vol.) **21**(4), 667–670.

Hamamci, N., Dursun, E., Ural, C. and Cakci, A. (1996) Calcitonin treatment in reflex sympathetic dystrophy: a preliminary study. *Brit. J. Clin. Prac.*, **50**(7), 373–375.

Hardy, M.A. and Hardy, S.G. (1997) Reflex sympathetic dystrophy: the clinician's perspective. *J. Hand Ther.*, **10**(2), 137–150.

Hooshmand, H. (1993) *Chronic Pain; Reflex Sympathetic Dystrophy, Prevention and Management*, CRC Press, Boca Raton, FL, pp. 13–26.

Kabeer, A.A. and Hardy, P.A. (1996) Long-term use of subarachnoid clonidine for analgesia in refractory reflex sympathetic dystrophy. Case report. *Reg. Anesth.*, **21**(3), 249–252.

Kaplan, R., Claudio, M., Kepes, E. and Gu, XF. (1996) Intravenous guanethidine in patients with reflex sympathetic dystrophy. *Acta Anaesth. Scand.*, **40**(10), 1216–1222.

King, J.H. and Nuss, S. (1993) Reflex sympathetic dystrophy treated by electroconvulsive therapy: intractable pain, depression, and bilateral electrode ECT. *Pain*, **55**(3), 393–396.

Kozin, F., McCarty, S.J., Sims, J. *et al.* (1976) The reflex sympathetic dystrophy syndrome. *Am. Gen. Med.*, **60**, 321–337.

Kumar, K., Nath, R.K. and Toth, C. (1997) Spinal cord stimulation is effective in the management of reflex sympathetic dystrophy. *Neurosurgery*, **40**(3), 503–508; discussion, 508–509.

Livingston, W.K. (1947) *Pain Mechanisms*, Macmillan, New York.

Manahan, A.P., Burkman, K.A., Malesker, M.A. and Benecke, G.W. (1993) Clinical observation on the use of topical nitroglycerin in the management of severe shoulder-hand syndrome. *Nebraska Med. J.*, **78**(4), 87–89.

Mellick, G.A. and Mellick, L.B. (1997) Reflex sympathetic dystrophy treated with gabapentine. *Arch. Phys. Med. Rehab.*, **78**(1), 98–105.

Mitchell, S.W., Morehouse, G.R. and Keen, W.W. (1864) *Gun Shot Wounds and Other Injuries of Nerves*, Lippincott, New York.

Mudun, A., Bursali, A., Oklu, T. *et al.* (1993) Scintigraphic evaluation of the effectiveness of intranasal calcitonin therapy in Sudeck's atrophy. *Nuc. Med. Comm.*, **14**(9), 805–809.

Muizelaar, J.P., Kleyer, M., Hertogs, I.A. and DeLange, D.C. (1997) Complex regional pain syndrome (reflex sympathetic dystrophy and causalgia): management with the calcium channel blocker nifedipine and/ or the alpha-sympathetic blocker phenoxybenzamine in 59 patients. *Clin. Neurol. Neurosurg.*, **99**(1), 26–30.

Poplawski, Z.J., Wiley, A.M. and Murray, J.F. (1983) Post traumatic dystrophy of the extremities; a review and trial of treatment. *J. Bone Joint Surg. (A)*, **65**, 642–654.

Ramamurthy, S., and Hoffman, J. (1995) Intravenous regional guanethidine in the treatment of reflex sympathetic dystrophy/causalgia: a randomised, double-blind study. Guanethidine Study Group. *Anesth. Analgesia*, **81**(4), 718–723.

Van Houdenhove, B., Vasquez, G. Onghena, P. *et al.* (1992) Etiopathogenesis of RSD; a review and biopsychosocial hypothesis. *Clin. J. Pain*, **8**, 300–306.

Walker, S.M. and Cousins, M.J. (1997) Complex regional pain syndromes: including 'reflex sympathetic dystrophy' and 'causalgia'. *Anaesthesia & Intensive Care*, **25**(2), 113–125.

Fibromyalgia

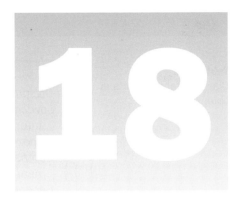

Fibromyalgia is a type of rheumatism which affects muscles and ligaments and is usually characterized by chronic musculo-skeletal symptoms of diffuse pain and tender points in the context of a normal laboratory and radiological examination. The current concept of fibromyalgia was described by Smythe and Moldofsky, who described certain musculoskeletal points which were very tender compared to the control (Smythe and Moldofsky, 1977). These musculoskeletal tender points were then verified by a few other studies in the 1980s (Yunus *et al.*, 1981; Campbell, 1983). The widely used criteria for the diagnosis of fibromyalgia is the one described by the American College of Rheumatology (Wolfe *et al.*, 1990).

To meet American College of Rheumatology 1990 diagnostic criteria for fibromyalgia, digital palpation with a force of about 4 kg should be performed. For a tender point to be considered 'positive' the subject must state that the palpation was painful. 'Tender' is not to be considered 'painful'. Widespread pain must have been present for at least 3 months. The presence of a second clinical disorder does not exclude the diagnosis of fibromyalgia. Pain on digital palpation must be present in at least 11 of the 18 tender point sites (Table 18.1). Some accept a diagnosis of fibromyalgia with fewer than 11 tender points if several associated symptoms, such as widespread pain, fatigue, morning stiffness, sleep disturbance, paresthesia and anxiety, are present.

Epidemiology

Fibromyalgia is more common in women. The peak age is between 30 and 50 years. In the American College of Rheumatology study, 89% of patients were female. The majority of these patients were Caucasian (93%), there being only 5% Hispanics and 1% Blacks.

The prevalence of fibromyalgia is about 2% in a family practice clinic, 5.7% in general medical clinic and about 14–20% in a rheumatology clinic.

Table 18.1
Classical tender points in fibromyalgia

Occiput – bilateral, at the suboccipital muscle insertions
Low cervical – bilateral, at the anterior aspects of the intertransverse spaces at C5–C7
Trapezius – bilateral, at the midpoint of the upper border
Supraspinatus – bilateral, at origins, above the scapula spine near the medial border
Second rib – bilateral, at the second costochondral junctions, just lateral to the junctions on upper surfaces
Lateral epicondyle – bilateral, 2 cm distal to the epicondyles
Gluteal – bilateral, in upper outer quadrants of buttocks in the anterior fold of the muscle
Greater trochanter – bilateral, posterior to the trochanteric prominence
Knee – bilateral, at the medial fat pad proximal to the joint line

Clinical features

The most common symptom of patients with fibromyalgia is chronic, diffuse pain arising from articular or non-articular areas. This pain usually begins in one location, the most common sites being the neck and shoulders, and with the passage of time it becomes generalized (Goldenberg, 1987).

Patients usually find it difficult to describe this pain and say it hurts all over. Their description of the nature of the pain also varies widely. Some patients describe it at a sharp pain, while others describe it as a diffuse or burning pain. The description of the intensity of the pain also varies.

One study assessed the sensitivity of pressure pain in different tissues in patients with fibromyalgia (Kosek, Ekholm and Hansson, 1995). The pressure pain thresholds were compared at a bony site, at a pure muscle site and at a site overlying the nerve. The site with the underlying nerve had the lowest pain threshold compared to the other two sites. As noted previously, this increased pain sensitivity in fibromyalgia patients was not altered by a local anaesthetic which led the authors to conclude that such pain is not dependent only on increased skin sensitivity.

The second most common symptom in patients with fibromyalgia is generalized fatigue. In one study (Wolfe, Hawley and Wilson, 1996), the factors predicting fatigue were pain and disturbance in sleep, as well as depression and tender point count. The fatigue in people with fibromyalgia is most notable first thing in the morning and also in the mid-afternoon. The intensity of fatigue varies and some patients become very tired after minor physical activities.

The other symptoms in patients with fibromyalgia include stiffness, which again is worse in the morning and after prolonged sitting. Some patients complain of headaches, which usually are occipital, though migraine is also more common in people with fibromyalgia.

People with fibromyalgia are also sometimes noted as having Raynaud's like symptoms, anxiety and depression. About 50% have symptoms suggestive of irritable bowel syndrome. Sleep disturbance is also common, patients sleeping 'lightly' and waking up early in the morning; some of them have difficulty in getting back to sleep.

Examination

The most notable examination finding in patients with fibromyalgia is the presence of multiple musculoskeletal tender points. Generally patients with fibromyalgia are apprehensive, but have no obvious features of systemic or articular abnormalities, though fibromyalgia can complicate a condition such as rheumatoid arthritis or osteoarthritis.

The best position to examine a patient with fibromyalgia is for him or her to be seated comfortably on the examination couch, so that the characteristic sites (Table 18.1) can be palpated. It is important not to apply excessive force at these points, since this can produce pain in most people. It is recommended that these sites should be palpated with thumb or forefinger, applying a pressure force of about 4 kg (Wolfe *et al.*, 1990).

The diagnostic utility of these tender points continues to generate heated debate. However, the criteria of at least 11 out of the 18 tender points are generally recommended for classification purposes, though they are in no way essential for the diagnosis of fibromyalgia.

Patients with fibromyalgia generally complain of muscle weakness. However, formal muscle power testing usually does not show any weakness. Patients sometimes complain of swelling of joints, but clinically there is no evidence of active synovitis. Paresthesias are reported by a majority of patients. However, neurological examination is normal.

Investigations

There are no specific biochemical or radiological tests for the diagnosis of fibromyalgia and basically it is a condition of exclusion. The minimal initial investigations should include a standard blood biochemistry and thyroid function test. Generally there is no need for extensive investigations, such as rheumatoid factor, antinuclear antibodies or serology for autoantibodies. Interestingly one study has reported a 10% prevalence of antinuclear antibodies in patients with fibromyalgia (Goldenberg, 1987). Unless there is strong evidence of an underlying serious pathology there is no need of muscle biopsy or scans such as MRI or an isotope bone scan.

Pathogenesis

The exact cause of fibromyalgia, as yet, is not known. The most common precipitating factors include a preceding flu-like viral illness, a physical or emotional trauma and sometimes withdrawal of medication, especially steroids. It is, however, common for patients with fibromyalgia to have no precipitating factors.

In view of the generalized fatigue, a possible role for muscle involvement has been extensively investigated over the past 10 years. So far no conclusive microscopic findings have been described. One study found an abnormal muscle metabolism in patients with fibromyalgia and concluded that these patients' fatigue is due to abnormalities of local tissue oxygenation at muscle tender sites (Lund, Bengdsson and Thorborg, 1986).

Sleep disturbance is common in patients with fibromyalgia and one study (Lario *et al.*, 1996) has demonstrated a small fall in the oxygen saturation of haemoglobin and arterial blood during overnight sleep.

Role of psychological factors

Pain is the most disabling symptom in patients with fibromyalgia. A recent study has suggested that the origin of this pain is primarily central rather than peripheral (Sorenson *et al.*, 1995). The authors gave intravenous morphine, lidocaine and ketamine to patients with fibromyalgia and measured the pain intensity, tolerance, muscle strength and muscle endurance. It was interesting to note that there was no response to morphine, but some reduction in pain intensity was noted after lidocaine. This led the authors to conclude that the tender points in fibromyalgia represent secondary hyperalgesia.

Management

Fibromyalgia is a complex condition, the exact aetiology of which remains unknown. The management of patients with fibromyalgia includes treatment with pharmaceuticals as well as non-medicinal treatment. Patient education constitutes an important part of management.

The pharmacological treatment for fibromyalgia is largely empirical and based on the pathophysiological abnormalities described above. Patients should be treated on an individual basis. The majority need medication to improve sleep and to diminish mood disturbances. They also need pain-killers to enhance peripheral and central analgesia.

Many patients find non-steroidal anti-inflammatory tablets of great help, though clinically and histologically there is no evidence of tissue inflammation. Those patients with predominant muscular symptoms usually respond better to an anti-inflammatory tablet. The improvement is usually short lasting and it is better to switch from one NSAID to another, keeping the dose as low as possible.

NSAIDs are usually not sufficient on their own to control symptoms of fibromyalgia, but they may have a synergistic effect when used in combination with an antidepressant, such as amitriptyline. Generally simple analgesics are of limited help in patients with fibromyalgia, but narcotics should not be used routinely in these patients.

The drugs most commonly used for mood disturbances and improved sleep pattern are amitriptyline and cyclobenzaprine. However, other tricyclics and different classes of central nervous system stimulating medications, including hydroxytryptophan have been found to be effective in a few studies. Tricyclics enhance stage four sleep and they are also known to have a central analgesic effect, owing to the increased brain serotonin activity as well as that of other neurogenic amines. Tricyclics are also known to have a peripheral analgesic effect. Benzodiazepines should not be used, as they block stage 4 sleep and may exacerbate fibromyalgia. Serotonin-specific reuptake inhibitors such as fluoxetine have not been effective except to symptomatically treat any associated depression.

Most of the central nervous system active medications have side-effects and, in particular, tricyclics can cause significant drowsiness and dry mouth. It is better to start a tricyclic at a very low dose, such as 5–10 mg of amitriptyline, 2–3 hours before bed time. The dose of amitriptyline should be increased gradually by about 5–10 mg at 2–3 week intervals. The majority of patients need between 25 and 50 mg at night; however, it is prudent to keep the dose as low as possible to avoid side-effects. Recently one study (Hrycag *et al.*, 1996) found significant improvement in pain, tender points and headaches in patients with fibromyalgia taking ondansetron, which is a 5 hydroxytryptamine receptor antagonist, compared to a placebo. There are at least four hydroxytryptamine receptor types and ondansatron is only a type 3 receptor antagonist.

Recently there have been a lot of studies on the role of non-medicinal treatment for fibromyalgia. Alternative medicines are used very commonly by patients with fibromyalgia (Table 18.2) (Goldenberg, 1997). In one study 21% of patients with fibromyalgia were taking some form of alternative medicine (Pioro-Boisset, Estaile and Fitzcharles, 1996). The most commonly used modalities are some form of local rubs and creams, including topical analgesics and counter-irritants. Some people get good benefit from vitamins and herbal products.

Patient satisfaction is also very high with other forms of treatment, including meditation, relaxation treatment with acupuncture, homeopathy, or reflexology. Many patients get good relief from a low-impact aerobic exercise programme, including activities such as swimming, fast walking, biking or water aerobics. The exercise programme needs to be tailored for the individual need, as patients with fibromyalgia generally perceive that their pain and fatigue increase with exercise. The role of other modalities of treatment, such as cardiovascular fitness training (McCain et al., 1988), EMG biofeedback (Ferraccioli, Ghiereli and Scita, 1987) and hypnotherapy (Haanen et al., 1991) has not been properly evaluated.

Table 18.2

Alternative medicine used by 80 patients with fibromyalgia

Therapy	Patients (%)	Satisfaction[a]
Over-the-counter items	70	6
Cream	50	
Vitamin	35	
Herbal products	29	
Spiritual practices	48	9
Prayers	41	
Meditation	38	
Relaxation	10	
Self-help group	6	
Spiritual healing	5	
Practitioners	40	8
Chiropractor	19	
Massage	10	
Acapuncture	8	
Homeopathy	4	
Reflexology	3	
Dietary modification	26	5
Addition to diet	20	
Subtraction from diet	25	

[a] Average of score; scale from 0 to 10, with 10 = most satisfied.
Reprinted, with kind permission, from Goldenberg (1997).

References

Campbell, S.N. (1983) Clinical characteristics of fibrositis; a blinded controlled study of symptoms and tender points. *Arthritis Rheum.*, **26**, 817–824.

Ferraccioli, G., Ghiereli, F. and Scita, S. (1987) EMG biofeedback training in fibromyalgia syndrome. *J. Rheumatol.*, **14**, 820–825.

Goldenberg, D.L. (1987) Fibromyalgia syndrome: an emerging, but controversial condition. *J. Am. Med. Assoc.*, **257**, 2782–2787.

Goldenberg, D.L. (1997) Fibromyalgia, chronic fatigue syndrome, and myofascial pain syndrome. *Curr. Opin. Rheum.*, **9**, 135–143.

Haanen, H.C.B., Hoenderbos, H.T.W., Van Romunde, L.K.J. *et al.* (1991) Controlled trial of hypnotherapy in the treatment of refractory fibromyalgia. *J. Rheumatol.*, **18**, 72–75.

Hrycag, P., Stratz, T., Mennet, B. *et al.* (1996) Pathogenetic aspects of responsiveness to ondansetron (5-hydroxytryptamine based type phase 3 receptor antagonist) in patients with primary fibromyalgia syndrome: a preliminary study. *J. Rheumatol.*, **23**, 1418–1423.

Kosek, E., Ekholm, J. and Hansson, B. (1995) Increased pressure pain sensibility in fibromyalgia patients is located deep to the skin, but not restricted to muscle tissue. *Pain*, 336–339.

Lario, B.A., Valdivielso, J.L.A., Lopez, J. *et al.* (1996) Fibromyalgia syndrome: overnight falls in arterial oxygen saturation. *Am. J. Med.*, **101**, 54–60.

Lund, N., Bengdsson, A. and Thorborg, P. (1986) Muscle tissue oxygen pressure in primary fibromyalgia. *Scand. J. Rheumatol.*, **15**, 165–173.

McCain, G.A., Bell, D.A., Mai, F.M. *et al.* (1988) A controlled study of the effects of a supervised cardiovascular fitness training programme on the manifestations of primary fibromyalgia. *Arthritis Rheum.*, **31**, 1135–1141.

Pioro-Boisset, M., Estaile, J.M. and Fitzcharles, M.A. (1986) Alternative medicine use in fibromyalgia syndrome. *Arthritis Rheum.*, **9**, 13–17.

Smythe, H.A. and Moldofsky, H. (1977) Two contributions to understanding of the fibrositis syndrome. *Bull. Rheum. Dis.*, **28**, 928–931.

Sorenson, J., Bengtsson, A., Backman, E. *et al.* (1995) Pain analysis in patients with fibromyalgia: effects of intravenous morphine, lidocaine and ketamine. *Scand. J. Rheumatol.*, **24**, 360–365.

Wolfe, F., Hawley, D.J. and Wilson, K. (1996) The prevalence and meanings of fatigue in rheumatic disease. *J. Rheumatol.*, **23**, 1407–1417.

Wolfe, F., Symthe, H.A., Yunus, M.B. *et al.* (1990) The American College of Rheumatology criteria for the classification of fibromyalgia: report of the multicentre criteria committee. *Arthritis Rheum.*, **33**, 160–172.

Yunus, M.B., Masai, A.T., Calabro, J.J. *et al.* (1981) Primary fibromyalgia (fibrositis): clinical history of 50 patients with matched normal control. *Semin. Arthritis Rheum.*, **11**, 151–171.

Intra-articular and para-articular corticosteroid injections

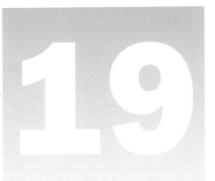

Corticosteroid injections are widely used in the treatment of patients with rheumatic disorders both intra-articularly and para-articularly. They are of great benefit to patients with inflammatory arthritis such as rheumatoid arthritis, inflammatory osteoarthritis and painful soft-tissue lesions.

The main indication for intra-articular injection is pain relief associated with an inflammatory arthritis and as an adjunct to systemic treatment. The natural course of an inflammatory arthritis such as rheumatoid arthritis is one of exacerbation and remission. If during the flare-up of rheumatoid arthritis two or three joints are predominantly affected, then it is worth aspirating and injecting the joints before deciding to increase systemic treatment, i.e. with a second-line disease-modifying agent. Corticosteroid injections into joints also help in mobilizing the inflamed joint by decreasing the pain and thereby preventing contracture formation, especially in children.

Raised intra-articular pressure due to an effusion also contributes to the pain and it is prudent to aspirate the joint before injection as this not only decreases the pressure and relieves pain, but also enhances the effect of the intra-articular corticosteroid. For a beginner, the easiest joints to inject are those with a large synovial cavity, such as the knee and shoulder joint or soft-tissue lesions that are easy to access, e.g. medial and lateral epicondylitis of the elbow (golfers and tennis elbow). There are certain joints that are difficult for the beginner to inject and are better injected by an expert under radiological control. These include spinal facet joints and the hips.

Soft-tissue lesions can be very painful and incapacitating and may be difficult to treat. Most of these lesions are self-limiting, but if there is no improvement after 4–6 weeks an intra-lesional corticosteroid injection may be helpful.

Contraindications

1. Intra-articular corticosteroids should not be used:
   - when there is an intra-articular or periarticular infection or septicaemia;
   - in patients with a known hypersensitivity to a previous injection;
   - in unstable joints.
2. Intra-articular corticosteroid should be used with caution in:
   - diabetics, as corticosteroids elevate the blood sugar level and can interfere with diabetic control for up to 2 to 3 weeks;
   - patients with established severe osteoporosis.

Commonly used intra-articular injections

There has been very little research comparing the efficacy of various intra-articular corticosteroids, but generally long-acting corticosteroids are more effective for intra-articular use because of low absorption from the synovial cavity. The most commonly used long-acting corticosteroid preparations are methylprednisolone acetate, with or without lignocaine, and triamcinolone hexacetonide and triamcinolone acetonide. Table 19.1 gives a list of commonly used corticosteroids for joint and soft-tissue injection.

Hydrocortisone acetate is relatively soluble and absorption from the joint is complete within 36 hours. It therefore has a rather weak anti-inflammatory action. Clinical improvement in a large inflamed rheumatoid joint after injection usually lasts for a few a days (Gray, Tenenbaum and Gottleib, 1981). The synthetic corticosteroids, including methylprednisolone acetate, triamcinolone acetonide and hexacetonide, on the other hand, are about five times more potent than hydrocortisone acetate because of

Table 19.1

Commonly used intra- and periarticular corticosteroid preparations

Preparation	Proprietary name (UK)
Hydrocortisone acetate	Hydrocortistab
Prednisolone acetate	Deltastab
Prednisolone phosphate	Codelsol
Dexamethasone acetate	
Methylprednisolone acetate	Depo Medrone with and without lignocaine
Triamcinolone hexacetonide	Lederspan 20 mg/ml
Triamcinolone acetonide	Kenalog 40 mg/ml
Dexamethasone phosphate	Decadron

their reduced solubility. Therefore their clinical effects can last for weeks or months.

There are no data available as to whether a particular joint responds well to a particular preparation. Generally if the patient does not respond to a single injection and provided that the diagnosis and technique were correct, it is worth trying an alternative preparation.

The long-acting insoluble synthetic corticosteroids can cause significant local tissue necrosis, such as subcutaneous fat atrophy, and therefore should be avoided in patients with periarticular and soft-tissue lesions. Skin atrophy can also occur following injection into a joint, as the corticosteroid can leak back, particularly in elderly patients.

Pharmacology

An inflamed joint is extremely vascular and therefore any preparation that is soluble or has a small molecule will diffuse into the circulation very quickly. Therefore, to achieve maximum sustained concentration of a drug in the synovium and synovial fluid, it is better to inject a preparation that has a relatively large molecule, is insoluble and is therefore absorbed slowly into the bloodstream. The absorption of corticosteroids from an inflamed joint is delayed by resting the injected joint for 24–48 hours, as this leads to a better clinical response.

Intra-articular or periarticular injection is a relatively safe procedure if done appropriately. Sepsis is always a concern and therefore it is very important to use an aseptic 'non touch' technique. The following steps should be taken to avoid introducing infection into a joint:

1. Wash your hands, preferably with an antiseptic solution. Gloves are generally not required.
2. Identify and mark the injection site.
3. Use pre-packed sterilized disposable needles and syringes. It is also better to use a single-dose ampoule for both corticosteroids and lignocaine.
4. It is also best not to inject air into the ampoule or the joint.
5. The skin should be thoroughly cleaned with isopropyl alcohol or similar antiseptic preparation.
6. After the injection site is clean use a non-touch technique. Never use your finger to guide the needle into the joint.
7. Apply a small sterilized gauze or an Elastoplast sticker after the injection.

Systemic absorption of the corticosteroid can cause suppression of the hypothalamic pituitary adrenal axis. However, after a single injection unwanted systemic side-effects are rare. Damage to a tendon or nerve is possible after a corticosteroid injection. This risk appears to be greatest for the Achilles tendon and to the long head of the biceps tendon and therefore these sites should not be routinely injected with long-acting corticosteroids.

PRACTICAL POINTS

Time interval when re-injecting same joints

There are no strict rules regarding the time interval between repeat injections at any particular site. However, it is generally better not to re-inject the same site within 3 weeks of the initial injection. The interval between repeat injections obviously depends on the clinical response, including duration of relief and patient's desire to have a repeat injection. The effect of intra-articular corticosteroids generally lasts longer in joints with a small synovial cavity, such as the small joints of the hands. On the other hand, in joints with a larger synovial cavity and those with an effusion, the clinical response may be of a shorter duration because the corticosteroid is more quickly absorbed into the circulation.

Frequency of intra-articular injection

It is better not to give an intra-articular injection more than three or four times a year into a particular joint. However, the soft-tissue lesions, such as the medial and lateral epicondylitis, usually respond with one or two corticosteroid injections given into the area of maximum tenderness.

Local anaesthesia before intra-articular injections

Some patients are very apprehensive and have a fear of injections. It is therefore always better to explain the procedure in detail, as this may avoid the need for skin and subcutaneous tissue anaesthesia with lignocaine. The pain threshold varies widely among individuals. Generally, however, injections into the large joints and those joints with an effusion are easier to perform than in those joints with smaller cavities.

Local anaesthesia can be achieved by a refrigerant spray, such as ethylchloride, followed by a 1% lignocaine intradermal injection, then waiting for 3–5 minutes before giving the intra-articular injection. Creams containing lignocaine and prilocaine are widely available, but these generally take a long time to exert a local anaesthetic effect.

Follow-up advice

After the injection the patient should be advised to rest the joint or soft tissue for about 24–48 hours. A follow-up appointment is usually needed after 3–4 weeks to reassess and to repeat the injection if required. It is also useful to have an information sheet about intra-articular injections (Figure

CORTICOSTEROIDS

(LOCAL INJECTION)

Figure 19.1
Patient information leaflet.

NAME:

1. WHY YOU ARE HAVING THIS INJECTION

This anti-inflammatory drug provides rapid relief of swelling, pain and stiffness for a severely inflamed single joint or tendon. It is particularly useful for a 'flare up' of inflammation in one or two joints.

2. HOW IS IT GIVEN?

Intra-articular steroids are injected by the doctor into the inflamed joint or around the tendon. It should be no more painful than having a blood sample. In some cases synovial fluid will be removed from the joint space before the injection is given.

3. HOW FAST DOES THE MEDICINE WORK?

Relief of symptoms should begin within 24 hours and may last for weeks, months or even longer. However, in some cases no relief is obtained; this does not mean they are not worth trying.

4. POINTS WORTH MENTIONING

- About one in five patients experience more **pain** for the first 36 hours after the injection. Anti-inflammatory painkillers during this time will help.
- Rarely, a small area of skin around the injection site may become permanently **pale in colour** and dimpled.
- **Rest** the injection area as much as possible for the first 48 hours following the injection. In the case of the shoulder, elbow, wrist or fingers, also try to avoid lifting heavy objects. If a weight-bearing joint is involved, i.e. hip, knee, ankle or foot, rest is even more important. Therefore, keep off it as much as possible for **48 hours**.
- **Infection** at the site of injection. This is very rare. However, you should watch for increased pain, heat and redness at the site of the injection 2 or 3 days afterwards. Report immediately to your GP if this occurs or telephone the department to see the doctor.
- **Diabetes**. Some diabetics may notice more sugar in the urine for up to 3 weeks after the injection of a large joint, e.g. knee or shoulder. This temporary increase does not usually require any change in diabetic treatment. If in doubt consult your GP.

19.1) for patients to read through before the injection and to take home afterwards.

INJECTION TECHNIQUE

The injection technique can be learned by reading the literature and knowing the exact anatomical landmarks. However, injections should not be given unless the clinician is familiar with the technique. The intra-articular and soft-tissue injection technique should be learned under the direct supervision of an experienced practitioner. There are certain helpful teaching manuals available (Golding 1991, 1992; Doherty *et al.*, 1992). The injection techniques for common conditions affecting different regions are as follows.

Hand

The metacarpophalangeal and proximal interphalangeal joints are commonly affected in rheumatoid arthritis, while the distal interphalangeal joints are more commonly affected by psoriatic arthritis. Osteoarthritis affects both proximal and distal interphalangeal joints and very commonly affects the first carpometacarpal joint.

The metacarpal and interphalangeal joints have a small synovial cavity and therefore it is best to use a small-gauge needle and about 5–10 mg of triamcinolone or an equivalent dose of another long-acting preparation. The joint line of the metacarpophalangeal joint could be palpated by asking the patient to flex the finger. The joint line lies about 1 cm distal to the crest of the knuckle. The MCP joint is best injected tangentially to the joint, just underneath the extensor expansion [Plate 1]. For the proximal [Plate 2] and distal interphalangeal joints the finger is flexed to about 45 degrees and slightly pulled distally. The joint is injected tangentially.

The first carpometacarpal joint is very commonly involved in osteoarthritis and can be very painful. The joint is injected from the lateral aspect near the abductor tendon [Plate 3] using a small-size needle and about 5–10 mg of triamcinolone.

The soft-tissue lesions, including tenosynovitis, can cause localized swelling or triggering of the fingers. Flexor tendon sheaths are injected just proximal to the metacarpal crease. The needle is advanced slowly until it finds a space, where the injection is given without resistance. For those who are not used to giving this injection it is best to check the position of the needle by asking the patient to flex his or her finger slowly; if correctly placed, there should be a very minimal movement of the needle.

Wrist

The soft-tissue lesions around the wrist include tenosynovitis of the flexor and extensor tendons as well as de Quervain's tenosynovitis and carpal tunnel syndrome. Rheumatoid and psoriatic arthritis both very commonly affect the wrist, while in the elderly chondrocalcinosis or pseudo-gout and osteoarthritis are usually the main culprit.

For carpal tunnel syndrome the injection site is just lateral to the midline underneath the tendon of palmaris longus. A fine-gauge needle is inserted into the tunnel at an angle of about 45 degrees to a depth of about 1 cm,

Plate 1 Technique for injecting metacarpophalangeal joint.

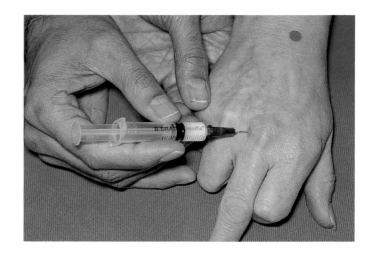

Plate 2 Technique for injecting proximal and distal interphalangeal joint.

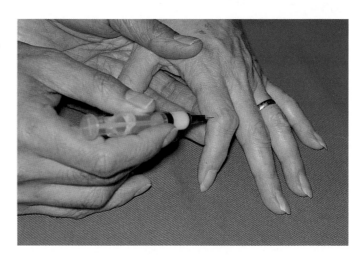

Plate 3 Technique for injecting first carpometacarpal joint.

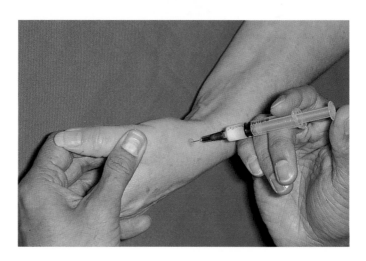

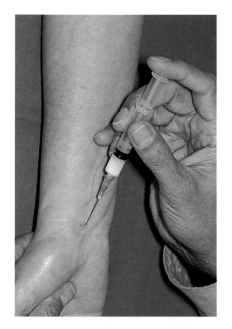

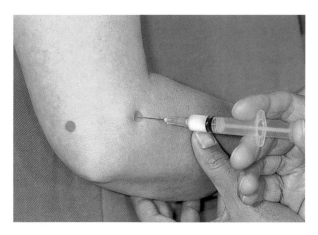

Plate 5 Technique for injecting Tennis elbow.

Plate 4 Technique for injecting carpal tunnel.

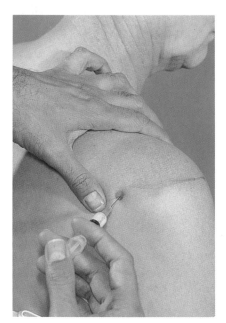

Plate 6 Posterior approach for injecting glenohumeral joint.

Plate 7 Technique for injecting sub-acromial space.

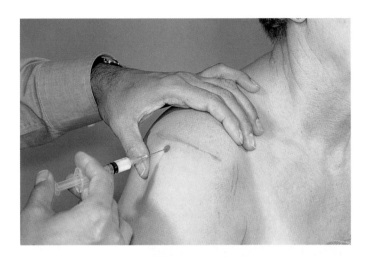

Plate 8 Technique for suprascapular nerve block.

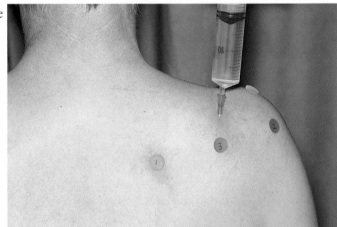

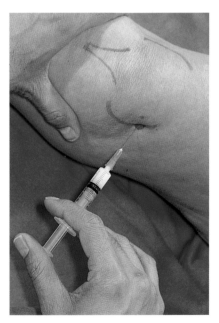

Plate 9 Technique for injecting knee by lateral approach.

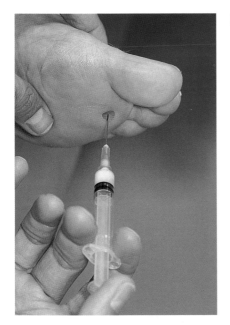

Plate 10 Technique for injecting metatarsophalangeal joint.

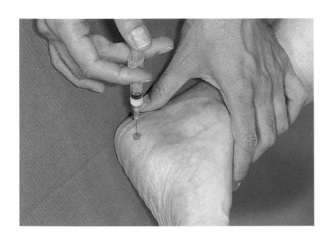

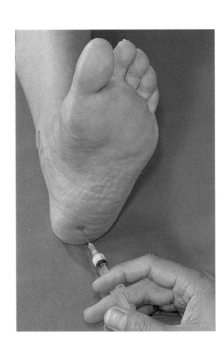

Plates 11 and 12 Technique for plantar fasciitis injection.

just medial to the palmaris longus tendon in the distal palmar crease [Plate 4]. Make sure there is no resistance to the injection. The usual dose is 5–10 mg of triamcinolone.

Tenosynovitis of the short extensor and the long abductor thumb tendons, also known as de Quervain's tenosynovitis, is usually very painful and interferes with pinching and gripping. In severe cases there is a palpable crepitus in the region of the tendon as the thumb is moved. Finklestein's test is usually positive. De Quervain's tenosynovitis is relatively easy to inject. The needle is inserted tangentially and a small amount of triamcinolone, i.e. 10–20 mg, along with 1–2 ml of 1% lignocaine is injected without resistance. Sometimes the examiner can feel the fluid as it moves along the tendon sheath. Chronic de Quervain's tenosynovitis usually requires surgical decompression.

The most commonly involved joints at the wrist are the radiocarpal joints and the lower radioulnar joints. For the radiocarpal joint the hand is slightly flexed so that it is easy to locate the T-shaped gap between the end of the radius and the lunate and scaphoid bones. About 20 mg of triamcinolone is injected at an angle of 60 degrees.

Elbow
Painful conditions around the elbow are quite common, particularly soft-tissue lesions, including lateral epicondylitis (tennis elbow), medial epicondylitis (golfer's elbow) and olecranon bursitis. Articular problems in isolation are rare at the elbow, but commonly occur in association with rheumatoid arthritis and sometimes with osteoarthritis.

Lateral epicondylitis
Lateral epicondylitis, also known as tennis elbow, is very common and affects about 1–3% of the population between the ages of 40 and 60. The pain is commonly localized over the lateral epicondyle and sometimes can radiate up and down the outer aspect of the elbow. Symptoms are usually made worse on resisted dorsiflexion of the wrist with the elbow in extension.

Many patients with soft-tissue lesions around the elbow settle spontaneously with rest and by taking a non-steroidal anti-inflammatory drug (NSAID) for a few weeks. However, in those patients with established epicondylitis a small amount of corticosteroid with or without local anaesthetic is usually helpful. Since the long-acting corticosteroids are insoluble and can cause skin depigmentation and subcutaneous fat atrophy, patients should be warned of this possibility or, preferably, given the first injection and a short-acting corticosteroid with 1% lignocaine.

For tennis elbow the injection is given at the site of maximum tenderness over the tenoperiosteal junction of the common extensor tendon [Plate 5].

The injection is therefore made under considerable pressure. It is better to infiltrate the area of maximum tenderness, which lies slightly distal to the epicondyle. After the injection advise the patient to avoid strenuous activity with the affected arm and to use an epicondlylitis clasp. Give a repeat injection 3–4 weeks after the initial injection if there is no significant improvement.

Medial epicondylitis

Medial epicondylitis, also known as golfer's elbow, is less common than lateral epicondylitis. Symptoms are similar to lateral epicondylitis, but localized medially at the common flexor tendon insertion at the medial epicondyle. Pain is made worse on resisted wrist flexion with the elbow in extension.

Medial epicondylitis is usually mild and responds to rest and a 2–3 week course of an NSAID. Some patients, however, require a corticosteroid injection. The technique for the injection of medial epicondylitis is the same as for lateral epicondylitis. One extra precaution concerns the proximity of the ulnar nerve, which lies in a groove just behind the medial epicondyle, and which should not be injected.

Olecranon bursitis

The olecranon bursa may be enlarged due to localized trauma or involved as part of a generalized arthritis in rheumatoid arthritis or gout. It is best aspirated with the elbow flexed at 90 degrees. If the overlying area is 'red hot' and painful, it is prudent to exclude infection and to assess the fluid for crystals. Once infection is excluded it is very easy to inject the olecranon bursa. The usual dose is 20 mg of methylprednisolone or an equivalent long-acting corticosteroid.

Elbow joint

There are two approaches to the elbow joint. The easiest one is the posterior approach. In this approach the elbow is flexed to about 90 degrees and comfortably supported on a pillow. Just above the olecranon process feel for the depression between the two halves of the triceps tendon. The injection site is just above the olecranon process at the olecranon fossa. It is not uncommon to find a small amount of fluid at this site. This should be aspirated and followed by an injection of 20–40 mg of methylprednisolone or an equivalent long-acting corticosteroid.

In the lateral approach, the patient's elbow is flexed to about 90 degrees. Locate the joint line by palpating the head of the radius and then gently pronating and supinating the patient's forearm. The needle is inserted tangentially from a supralateral position.

Shoulder

Painful shoulder is very common, particularly in the elderly. Shoulder problems are usually due to soft-tissue lesions and true osteoarthritis of the glenohumeral joint is rare. Common shoulder problems include capsulitis (frozen shoulder), rotator cuff tendonitis with impingement syndrome, and osteoarthritis of the glenohumeral and acromioclavicular joint.

Glenohumeral joint

The glenohumeral joint can be approached both anteriorly and posteriorly. The posterior approach is much easier and carries less risk.

For the posterior approach the patient is seated comfortably in a chair and advised to relax the shoulder girdle muscles. The injection site is easy to find by initially locating the posterior margin of the acromion and with the forefinger locating the coracoid process, which lies anteriorly. The injection site is 1 cm infromedial to the posterior angle of the acromion with needle pointing towards the outer site of the coracoid process [Plate 6]. A long-acting corticosteroid, such as methylprednisolone 40 mg or equivalent with or without lignocaine, is injected.

The anterior approach is more difficult. For this the patient lies supine or semi-reclined with the forearm laid across the abdomen, i.e. the shoulder is partially internally rotated. In this position it is easy to feel the joint line, which lies lateral to the coracoid process. The injection is given slightly infrolateral to the coracoid process.

Acromioclavicular joint

This is a small joint that is easy to identify. A small-gauge needle is used and the joint can be approached either inferiorly or anterosuperiorly. Owing to the small joint cavity, it is rarely possible to inject more than 0.5 ml of fluid into this joint.

Subacromial space

This is the site for a local corticosteroid injection to treat rotator cuff tendonitis and impingement and subacromial bursitis. It is important to seat the patient comfortably with relaxed shoulder girdle muscles so that the gap between the acromion and the head of humerus can be easily palpated.

The best approach to the subacromial space is laterally. First palpate the most lateral point of the acromion, from where it is easy to access the subacromial space from either a lateral or a posterolateral approach. The needle is aimed medially and slightly upwards to avoid injecting into the rotator cuff tendon [Plate 7].

Bicipital tendonitis

In bicipital tendonitis the pain is located anteriorly over the shoulder. Bicipital tendonitis usually occurs in association with rotator cuff impingement or tendonitis. Treatment for the rotator cuff impingement usually eases the symptoms of bicipital tendonitis as well.

It is easy to inject the bicipital groove by resting the patient in a semi-inclined position with the arm slightly externally rotated, the shoulder extended and the elbow flexed. The injection is given into the bicipital groove. Care should be taken not to inject the tendon itself, which can lead to rupture. A small amount of a short-acting corticosteroid is injected into the site of maximum tenderness.

Suprascapular nerve block

Shoulder pain can become chronic and disabling and may not respond to the conventional treatment of an NSAID, physiotherapy and an intra-articular intralesional injection. Those patients not suitable for surgery may be candidates for suprascapular nerve block. It is a relatively safe and easy technique which has been successfully used in the treatment of chronic shoulder pain from soft-tissue lesions or arthritis of the glenohumeral joint (Vecchio, Adebajo and Hazelman, 1993; Dangoisse, Wilson and Glynn, 1994).

The injection site is about 2–3 cm above and lateral to a point defined by the bisection of two lines, one along the spine of the scapula posteriorly and the other from the inferior angle of the scapula vertically upwards. The needle is inserted in an inward, forward and downward direction towards the suprascapular notch [Plate 8].

The risk of pneumothorax is reduced by asking the patient to place the ipsilateral hand on the opposite shoulder which elevates the scapula and moves it away from the thoracic wall. It is a relatively safe procedure which can be carried out in outpatients, though, ideally, it is better to do it under radiological control.

Injection of hip and soft tissue around the hip joint

Hip joint

The hip joint is a true ball-and-socket joint which lies quite deep and it is therefore difficult to feel the joint line. It is better to inject the hip joint under fluoroscopic guidance. The patient lies with hips slightly flexed and externally rotated. The needle is inserted two fingers width lateral to the femoral artery just below the inguinal ligament at the intersection of the vertical line drawn from the anterior superior iliac spine and a horizontal line drawn from the greater trochanter.

Trochanteric bursitis

This is the commonest cause of pain around the hip region. The bursa is usually not palpable unless partly inflamed or distended. The pain due to trochanteric bursitis is localized over the lateral aspect of the hip and thigh.

Injection for trochanteric bursitis is relatively easy. The patient lies with the affected side uppermost and flexed. The unaffected hip is extended while the uppermost thigh is allowed to fall into slight adduction. It is easy to identify the site of maximum tenderness over the trochanteric prominence. A 20 gauge needle is inserted vertically until it touches the bone, when it is slightly withdrawn and the patient is injected with a long-acting corticosteroid and local anaesthetic. Injection is given in several directions along the affected area, followed by gentle massage to help distribute the drug uniformly over a wider area.

Ischiogluteal bursitis

It is easy to locate the site of maximum tenderness in ischiogluteal bursitis. The patient is rested on the examination couch, lying on one side with hips slightly flexed. The area of maximum tenderness is infiltrated with a mixture of a long-acting corticosteroid and a local anaesthetic. The sciatic nerve lies just lateral to the bursa and care should be taken not to inject it.

Meralgia paraesthetica

This is an entrapment neuropathy due to compression of the lateral cutaneous nerve of the thigh as it passes under the inguinal ligament. First locate the tender spot at the site where the lateral cutaneous nerve of the thigh penetrates the fascia of the upper thigh about 10 cm below the anterior superior iliac crest. This site is then infiltrated with a mixture of a long-acting corticosteroid and 3–5 ml of 1% lignocaine.

Adductor tendonitis

Adductor tendonitis is common in athletes. The critical site of the pain is in the groin and inner aspect of thigh, which is made worse on resisted adduction of the hip. The majority of patients respond with rest and physiotherapy, including stretching exercises, ultrasound and a course of an NSAID.

Treatment, however, differs from site to site; if only the muscle belly is affected, it usually responds to massage with or without local anaesthetic. Where the lesion is at the tenoperiosteal junction either massage or a 20 mg corticosteroid injection with 1 or 2 ml of 1% lignocaine is infiltrated to the tender area in a series of droplets, followed by massage to distribute the drug over a wider area.

Knee joint

The knee joint is quite superficial, has a large synovial cavity and is therefore relatively easy to inject. It is usually injected either by a lateral retropatellar or medial retropatellar approach; however, it can also be injected from a suprapatellar or anterior approach.

For both the medial and lateral approach the patient lies supine with the knee extended. The injection site is at the junction of the middle and upper third of the patella on either site. When there is an effusion the approach to the knee is made easier by increasing the gap between the patella and the femur. Alternatively this gap can be increased manually by slightly pushing the patella laterally.

An 18–21 gauge needle is introduced at the junction of upper and middle third with the needle pointing slightly upwards toward the suprapatellar pouch [Plate 9]. The usual dose is 40 mg of methylprednisolone or an equivalent dose of a long-acting corticosteroid. The anterior approach is not commonly used. In this method the knee is first flexed to about 90 degrees and the needle is then inserted just lateral to the patellar tendon at a slightly upward direction into the intercondylar fossa.

Swellings in the popliteal region are common and can occur at any age. A large popliteal cyst can interfere with knee movement and may need surgical excision. Aspiration of the popliteal cyst is quite easy, though fluid usually reaccumulates after aspiration and injection of corticosteroids.

Soft tissue lesions, such as bursitis and tendonitis, are quite common around the knees. For pre-patella bursitis the needle is inserted at the point of maximum fluctuation. Fluid is aspirated and the bursa can be injected, if infection is excluded, with a small amount of corticosteroid. The deep infrapatellar bursa can be approached from either the lateral or the medial aspect. The needle is directed deep to the patellar ligament just proximal at its insertion to the tibial tubercle.

Other soft-tissue lesions around the knee, such as pre-patellar tendonitis, iliotibial band friction syndrome and pain localized to the insertion of the medial or lateral collateral ligament of the knee, usually respond to rest and a course of an NSAID. Resistant cases, however, need a steroid injection into the tender site.

Ankle and foot

Ankle joint

The ankle joint is best approached anteriorly. The injection site is just lateral to the tibialis anterior tendon, which is easy to identify when the patient dorsiflexes the foot. The space immediately lateral to the tibialis anterior tendon, i.e. between the tibia and the talus is the point of entry where the needle is injected tangentially to the curve of the talus.

Sub-talar joint

This joint is rather difficult to inject. The patient is seated comfortably and the point of entry is lateral to the junction of a horizontal line drawn 2.5 cm above the end of the lateral malleolus and a vertical line 1 cm from the posterior border of the shaft of the fibula.

Metatarsophalangeal joints

The metatarsophalangeal joint has small synovial cavity, but can be entered by a dorsolateral or dorsomedial approach [Plate 10]. Slight distal traction of the affected toe usually helps in localizing the joint line.

Plantar fasciitis

The best option is to locate the point of maximum tenderness, which can then be injected using a medial approach if the skin is relatively thin [Plate 11] or alternatively directly through the plantar surface [Plate 12]. The injection is made close to the bony surface.

Achilles bursitis

The best approach for the Achilles bursitis is from lateral side. The injection site is very close to the Achilles tendon, which should not be injected. The entry point is just above the top of the calcaneum, where the needle is directed medially and slightly downwards into the bursa.

Morton's neuroma

This is a painful lesion which usually lies between either the second and third or the third and fourth toes. The site of injection is the point of maximum tenderness, which is injected directly with a mixture of a small amount of a long-acting corticosteroid and a local anaesthetic.

Tibialis posterior tendonitis

The tibialis posterior tendon sheath is often swollen in rheumatoid arthritis and causes pain which can be relieved by a local cortisone injection. The tendon sheath is entered tangentially, directing the needle proximally just below and behind the medial malleolus. A correctly placed injection distends the tendon sheath, which can be felt as it spreads proximally.

Tarsal tunnel syndrome

The injection site for tarsal tunnel syndrome is under the flexor retinaculum between the medial malleolus and the calcaneus.

Temporomandibular joint

The temporomandibular joint is easy to inject and usually responds to a local injection. The patient is seated in a reclining position with a head support. The joint line is easily felt by placing the finger in front of the tragus, and by asking the patient to open and close the mouth, the condyle of the mandible can be felt. The injection site is overlying the joint line and the needle is directed slightly upwards and a small amount of hydrocortisone or a long-acting corticosteroid is injected into the joint.

Caudal epidural injection

Caudal epidural injection is a safe technique and can be given to an outpatient. The patient is rested prone with buttocks exposed and it is helpful to put a small pillow under the abdomen to raise the pelvis. Identify the injection site at the sacral hiatus and mark it with a ballpoint pen. The skin in the lower sacrum and the intergluteal cleft is then sterilized. The operator can sit or stand to the left of patient. The skin is anaesthetized by 2% lignocaine. For the epidural an ordinary lumbar-puncture needle is passed through the anaesthetic area of the skin and into the intercornual space at an angle of about 45 degrees pointing upwards. As the needle passes through the sacral hiatus there is a feeling of give when the needle should be passed for a further 3–4 cm.

In most patients the thecal sac ends at the lower level of the first sacral vertebra. It is very important to abandon the procedure if cerebrospinal fluid escapes from the epidural needle, suggesting damage to the dura mater. The procedure should then be postponed for at least 3 days to allow the puncture to heal.

A mixture of 20–50 ml of fluid containing 0.25–0.5% marcaine with 80–120 mg of methylprednisolone acetate is injected very slowly and is given over a period of 5–10 minutes. To make sure the injection is given into the sacral hiatus the operative's left hand rests on the sacrum in order to detect any bulge appearing due to fluid being injected into subcutaneous tissue.

After the injection the patient should be observed for 30–60 minutes for any untoward side-effects. The author's practice is to observe the patient for about 2 hours, with half hourly pulse and blood pressure checks.

References

Dangiosse, M.J., Wilson, D.J. and Glynn, C.J. (1994) MRI and clinical study of an easy and safe technique of suprascapular nerve blockade. *Acta Anaes. Belgica*, 45(2), 49–54.

Doherty, M., Hazelman, B.L., Hutton, C.W. *et al.* (1992) *Rheumatology Examination and Injection Techniques*, W.B. Saunders, London.

Golding, D.N. (1991) Local corticosteroid injections. Part I: General aspects and the upper limb. Practical problems. *Reports on Rheumatic Diseases (Series 2)*, No 19, Arthritis and Rheumatism Council.

Golding, D.N. (1992) Local corticosteroid injections. Part II: The lower limb. Practical problems. *Reports on Rheumatic Diseases (Series 2)*, No 20. Arthritis and Rheumatism Council.

Gray, R.G., Tenenbaum, J. and Gottleib N.L. (1981) Local corticosteroid injection treatment in rheumatic disorders. *Semin. Arthritis Rheum.*, **10**, 231–254.

Vecchio, P.C, Adebajo, A.O. and Hazelman, B.L. (1993) Suprascapular nerve block for persistent cuff lesions. *J. Rheumatol.*, **20**(3), 453–455.

Index